MAKEUP
ARTIST

LIP CHARTS

FROM THE BEAUTY STUDIO COLLECTION

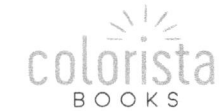

colorista
BOOKS

www.coloristabooks.com

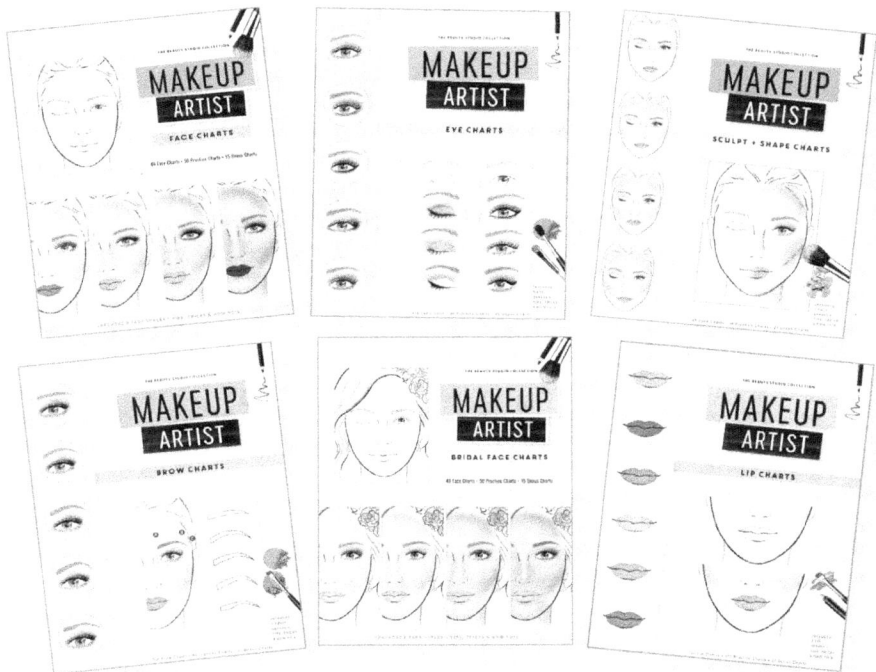

Contents

LIP CHARTS

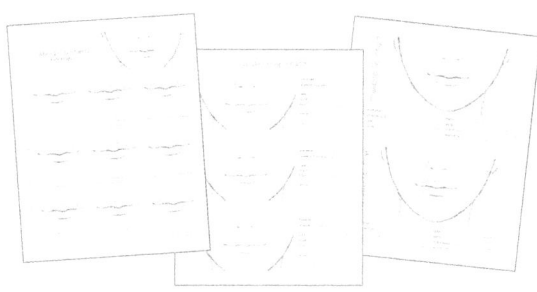

126 total eye charts - 21 of each shape.

BONUS MAKEUP CHARTS

Sample makeup charts from other books in the Beauty Studio Collection!

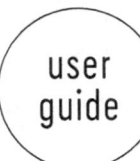
GETTING STARTED

This book contains practice charts, makeup charts and bonus makeup charts for hours of coloring fun! Follow the User Guide to discover tips, techniques, and how-to's to customize your makeup looks like a pro!

Color & customize your makeup charts with colored pencils, markers, crayons, even real makeup! Makeup charts include product/color logs so you can easily keep track of what you use for each look.

COLORING WITH MAKEUP

Dry makeup formulas such as powder eyeshadow, blush, bronzer & flesh-tone face powders blend easily on paper. An advantage of powder, is that it can be removed with an eraser. White erasers are recommended over colored ones as they are less likely to stain.

You may find cream & liquid products diffcult to use as they tend to apply blotchy & can leave oil stains. However, is possible to use these types of products if you apply them in thin layers. See '**Pro Tips + Tricks**', to learn more about cream & liquid application techniques.

ABOUT PAPER TEXTURE

Paper texture or "tooth" is about how the surface of paper feels. The more tooth paper has, the rougher it will feel because it has lots of tiny bumps & grooves. Makeup face charts within this book are printed on paper with little tooth, giving it a fairly smooth texture. Now, depending on your choice of coloring material(s), you may find that some products adhere better than others.

If certain products/colors aren't applying as vibrant as you would like, consider adding some tooth to the paper. An easy ways to do this is with texture hairspray (aerosol) - simply mist the surface of the paper with a thin layer and let dry.

Another way to add tooth is with clear gesso paste.* Apply a thin even layer with a wide synthetic paint brush and let dry. Rinse brush with water immediately after use. If paper feels too gritty, gently smooth surface with fine sandpaper.

* Clear Gesso by Liquitex, Artist's Acrylic or Dina Wakley is recommended.

MAKEUP APPLICATION TOOLS

When it comes to applying makeup on a chart, you'll find that smaller brushes offer more control over placement & blending. The most useful eye brushes include:

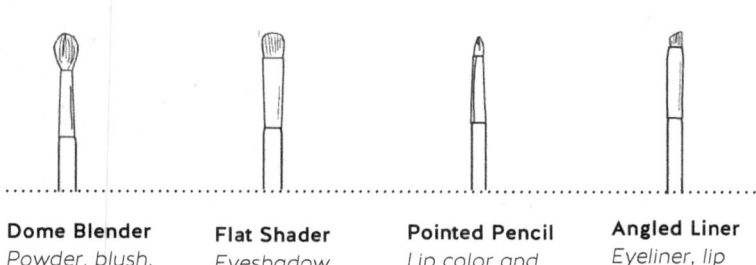

Dome Blender
Powder, blush, bronzer, contour and highlight

Flat Shader
Eyeshadow and contour

Pointed Pencil
Lip color and defining eyes

Angled Liner
Eyeliner, lip liner & defining brows

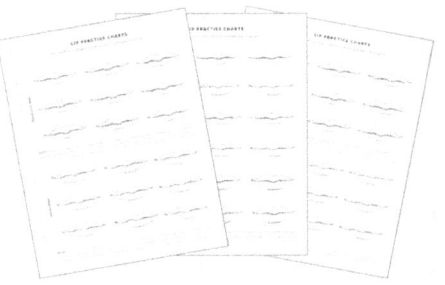

Build your sills with practice charts

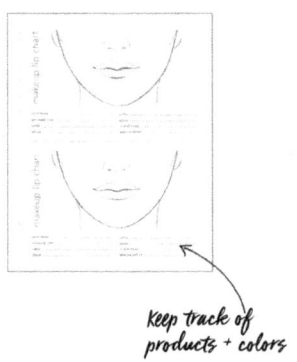

keep track of products + colors

HOW TO BUILD A PORTFOLIO

Create your own makeup portfolio to showcase your skills & looks. All you'll need are scissors, 8.5" x 11" (3-ring) binder & clear protective sleeves. Cut along dashed line to remove makeup chart from book & put in protective sleeve.

Use binder tab dividers to categorize & organize looks by makeup styles (day, night, bridal, dramatic, smokey eyes, etc..) and/or makeup looks for various skintones (fair, light, med, tan, dark).

Alternatively, you can leave makeup charts in book and use sticky note tab labels to catergorize and organize.

Adding Skincolor

• Add any shade of skin color to a makeup chart with flesh-tone face powder and a dome blender brush.

• For smooth even results, pick up powder with brush then dab on back of hand to distribute powder evenly into the bristles. Use light circular motions to color in "skin". Repeat until you have reached your desired shade.

• Avoid whites of eyes as you shade in skin. If any makeup gets onto the eyes, use a white eraser to remove it. Alternatively, you can mask the eyeballs before you color the skin with removable tape or a thin coat of clear nail polish.

Powder Makeup

For smooth application - pick up powder with brush & dab on back of hand to distribute evenly into the bristles. Use small circular motions when blending color on paper. Repeat until you reach desired shade.

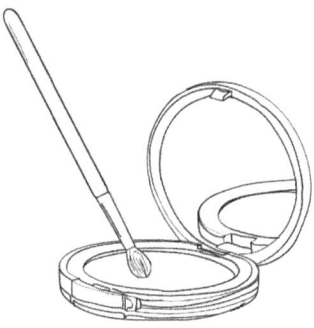

Cream + Liquid Makeup

The key to achieving the best results with cream & liquid makeup is to apply in thin layers.

HOW TO APPLY CREAMS + LIQUIDS:

1. Put a little makeup on back of your hand.

2. Pick up makeup with dome blender brush.

3. Use dabbing & circular motions on back of hand to evenly distribute makeup into the bristles.

4. Apply color on paper with gentle swiping & circular motions.

5. Repeat steps 1-4 until you reach desired shade.

Eye Enhancements

• For a realistic eye color effect mix blue, green or orange eyeshadow with a bit of brown and/or grey eyeshadow. Fill in eye color with a pointed pencil brush.

• Add a coat of clear shiny nail polish over eye color for a natural glossy effect.

• Keep eraser handy to remove makeup that gets on whites of eyes.

Eyeliner Tips

• Apply a clear nail polish (matte or glossy top coat) over creamy eye pencils or liquid eyeliner to seal & keep from smudging.

• Substitute creamy eyeliner with products that dry and won't smudge. China Markers (by Dixon or Sharpie) make a great substitute for eye pencils. Fine-point permanent markers (by Sharpie) or ink (used with dip pen) can give you the look of rich liquid liner.

• Create the look of white eyeliner with liquid white-out corrector (look for it in a fine-point pen by BIC or Sharpie).

• Dark eyeshadow can be used in place of pencil & liquid eyeliners. For sharp crisp lines, apply with an angled liner brush. For a soft & smokey effect, line eyes with a pointed pencil brush.

Sparkle Effect

Glitter is a fun & easy way to add a touch of glitz & glam to your makeup looks.

HOW TO APPLY GLITTER:

1. Use brush or finger to spread an even layer of clear school or craft glue onto makeup chart (applying glue with tool will provide more even coverage).
2. Pour glitter over glue.
3. Hold makeup chart upright and tap to get rid of excess glitter. Be sure to lay paper under makeup chart to catch extra glitter.

Metallic Pigments

Highly-reflective metallic finishes are a great way to add a dimension and shine to makeup charts. For best results, use metallic pigments in powder form (eyeshadow, loose pigment, etc...). For application of liquid metallic makeup see tip on **'Cream + Liquid Makeup'**.

HOW TO APPLY METALLIC PIGMENTS:

1. Pick up powder on flat shader brush.
2. Lightly mist with water until slightly damp.
3. Distribute powder & water into the bristles by gently dabbing on the back of your hand.
4. Apply on paper with dabbing/pressing motions & let dry.
5. Use dry dome blender brush & metallic powder to blur any hard lines (use small circular motions along edges to create a seamless blend).

Cleaning Brushes

Using the same brush for multiple applications can easily lead to "muddy" colors. A simple way to avoid this is with a quick "dry cleaning" in between applications to remove color residue left on bristles. Simply wipe your brush on a damp baby wipe (or damp paper towel with a little baby shampoo lather). Then wipe bristles on a dry paper towel to remove excess moisture.

Adding Highlights

Highlights give face charts a pro look by adding dimension. Highlights can be easily achieved with the 'Reverse Highlighting Technique' - simply add color to makeup chart then use an eraser to remove color where you want highlights to be.

Lip Color

• Substitute creamy lip products with powder eyeshadow or colored pencils.

• Real lipgloss is not recommended for makeup charts as it can easily smear. A great substitute for lip gloss is shiny clear nail polish. Apply a coat of clear shiny nail polish over lips for glossy effect.

• Create your own custom tinted "lipgloss" by mixing clear nail polish & powder eyeshadow.

• To create a tinted gloss in a shade similar to real lips, mix clear nail polish with peachy-mauve eyeshadow or blush. Add matte white eyeshadow to lighten and make more opaque.

HOW TO MAKE TINTED LIPGLOSS:

1. Cut a square piece of foil (about 4 x 4 inches). Gently push a finger into the center of foil to create a bowl.

2. Pour clear nail polish in bowl until 1/4 - 1/2 full.

3. Scrap a little bit of eyeshadow into bowl using needle or toothpick.

4. Mix powder & polish well with applicator brush.

5. Test color on white piece of scrap paper. Keep adding eyeshadow & testing until you reach desired shade. If color is too dark, add more clear polish or white eyeshadow.

6. Apply color to lips immediatley.
Clean applicator brush with nail polish remover before dipping back into polish bottle.

Set and Seal

Protect & preserve completed face charts from moisture, fading and smearing with an 'artist fixative' or 'paper protectant' spray. You will need a well-ventilated area when using these types of products - please follow directions carefully!
*Krylon Preserve It Matte' is recommended.

LIP ENHANCEMENTS

This book contains various lip shapes from thin to extra-full. Although lip enchancements are generally meant for thinner lips, the following techniques can be used to add volume & fullness to any lip shape. Use the lip practice charts to help you build your skills!

Over-lining

WHAT YOU NEED

☐ Pencil ☐ Eraser ☐ Angled liner brush ☐ Pencil brush
☐ Lip liner ☐ Lip color

The key to achieving the most natural results with over-lining, is to avoid lining outside the natural lip line at the corners of the mouth. Over-lining the corners creates a "clown-mouth" effect.

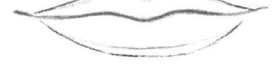

1. Sketch new lipline slightly above center of upper or lower lip. Follow shape of lip until you are about 1/2 way to corner of mouth then meet up with natural lip line. Keep eraser handy to correct mistakes.

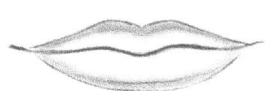

2. Define new lip line by going over it with lip-liner & angled liner brush. Fill in space between lips & new lip line. Also apply to corners of lips.

3. Add lip color to pencil brush. Fill in blank area of lips with lip color. Use soft circluar motions where liner meets color for a seamless blend.

Highlight + Shade

WHAT YOU NEED

☐ Face powder ☐ Contour powder
☐ Lipcolor ☐ Pencil brush

OUTSIDE OF LIPS

1. Add skin color to face (**see Pro Tips + Tricks**).
2. Use an eraser to remove color along cupid's bow (V part of the upper lip) & sides of lower lip.
3. Apply shading under the lower lip with pencil brush & contour powder.

INSIDE OF LIPS

1. Fill in lips with your choice of color.
2. Use an eraser to remove color from the bow of the upper lip & along the center of bottom lip.
3. Blur any hard edges left from eraser with pencil brush (use small circular motions create a seamless transition from lip color to reflection areas).

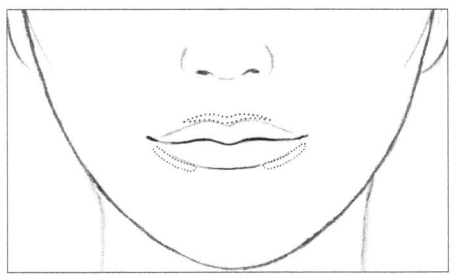

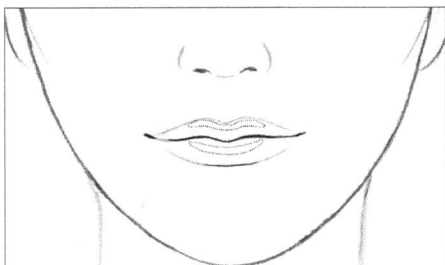

PRO LIP EFFECTS

Nude Lips

WHAT YOU NEED
- ☐ Pencil brush ☐ Nude lipcolor
- ☐ Lipliner ☐ Eraser

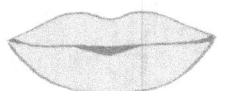

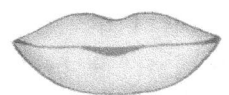

1. Apply nude color to entire lips with pencil brush.

2. Apply liner to outer edge of lips with pencil brush. Use small circular motions where dark & light meet to create a seamless blend.

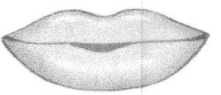

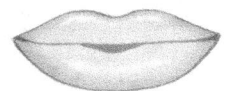

3. Use eraser to add highlights on upper & bottom lip.

4. Optional: Apply coat of shiny clear polish for a glossy finish.

Ombre Lips

WHAT YOU NEED
- ☐ Pencil brush ☐ Angled liner brush
- ☐ Light lipcolor ☐ Dark lipcolor

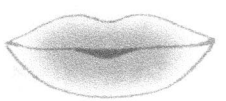

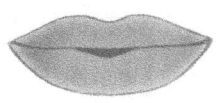

1. Apply lightest color to center of lips with pencil brush (concentrate the most color in the center & gradually fade out.)

2. Apply darkest color on outer edges of lips with pencil brush. Use small circular motions where dark meets light to create a seamless blend.

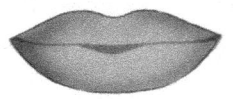

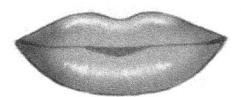

3. Add more dark color to intensify outer edges of lips. Apply with angled liner brush - use soft strokes to avoid harsh lines.

4. Optional: For a glossy ombre, use eraser to add highlights & apply coat of shiny clear polish.

PRO TIPS

- *See 'Pro Tips + Tricks' for how-to on mixing your own tinted lipgloss.*
- *When using light nude shades on dark skintones, use a brown lip liner to create a seamless transition from skin to lips.*
- *If a nude lip is too pale, tone it down with tinted lipgloss in a shade similar to natural lips (neutral peachy-mauve).*

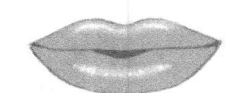

Glossy Lips

For full plump lips with a high-shine finish.

WHAT YOU NEED:
Lip color, pencil brush, eraser, clear shiny nail polish

HOW TO APPLY:
1. Color in lips with pencil brush.
2. Add reflection on upper & bottom lip with eraser.
3. Apply a coat of polish for a glossy finish.

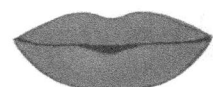

Ombre Lips

Achieve rich velvety texture without the mess of matte liquid lipstick.

WHAT YOU NEED:
Marker (choice of lipcolor) matte eyeshadow (same shade as lipcolor), pencil brush

HOW TO APPLY:
1. Fill in lips with marker
2. Use pencil brush to apply matte eyeshadow over marker.

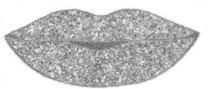

Glitter Lips

Add a touch of glitz & glam to your looks with sparkle.

WHAT YOU NEED:
Glitter, clear school glue*, finger or brush to apply glue, clear shiny nail polish

HOW TO APPLY:
1. Spread thin layer of glue on lips.
2. Pour glitter on lips.
3. Remove excess glitter.
4. Seal glitter with coat of polish.

* Clear glue works best with glitter as white glue can dry cloudy & dull shine.

LIP PRACTICE CHARTS

Use templates to design looks and practice application techniques.

Thin

Thin-upper

Thin-lower

Medium

Full

Extra-full

NOTES_____

_____

_____

LIP PRACTICE CHARTS

Use templates to design looks and practice application techniques.

Thin Lip Shape

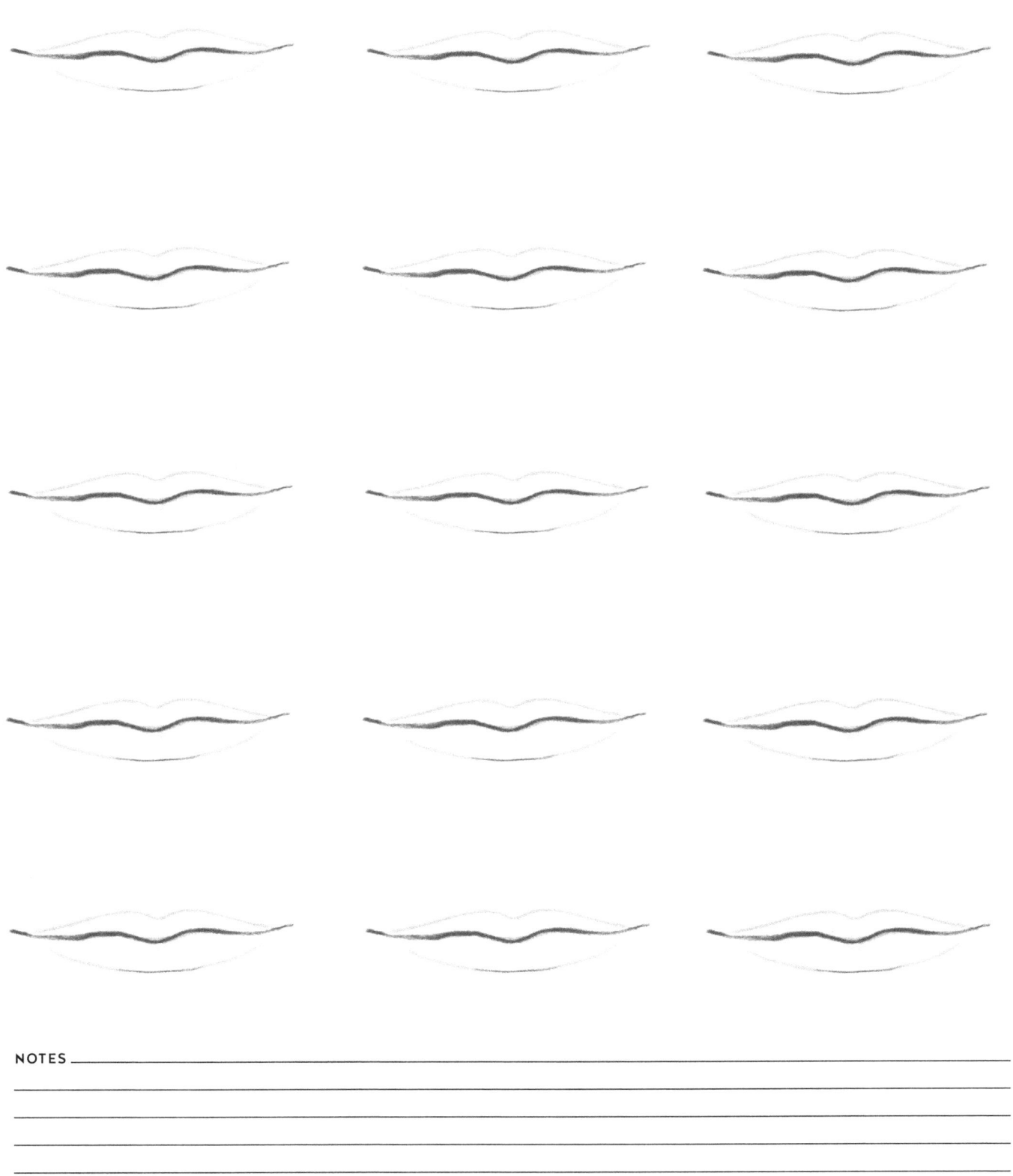

NOTES _____

_____

_____

_____

_____

LIP PRACTICE CHARTS

Use templates to design looks and practice application techniques.

Thin-upper Lip Shape

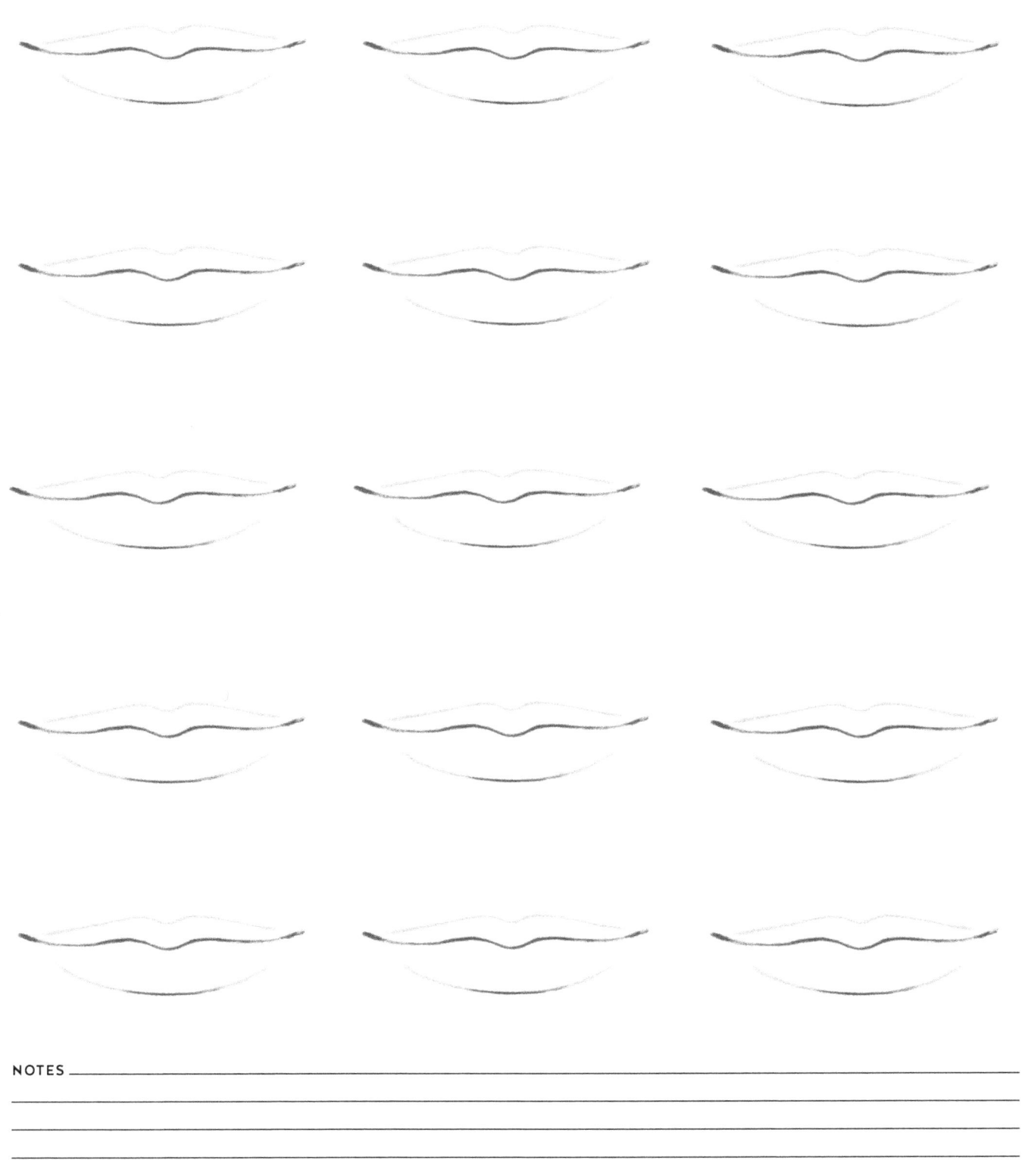

NOTES _____

_____

_____

_____

_____

LIP PRACTICE CHARTS

Use templates to design looks and practice application techniques.

Thin-lower Lip Shape

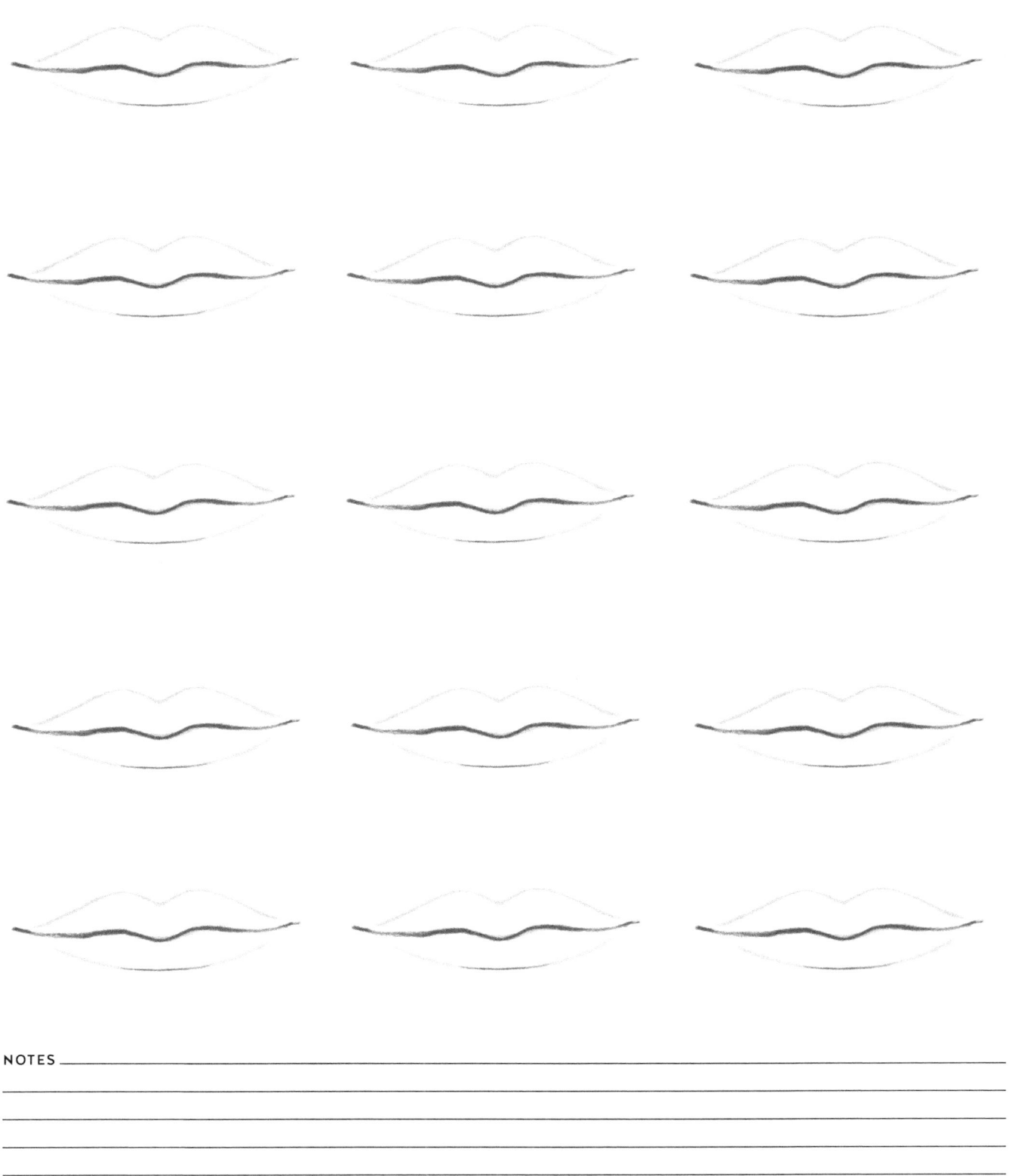

NOTES _____
_____
_____
_____
_____

LIP PRACTICE CHARTS

Use templates to design looks and practice application techniques.

Medium Lip Shape

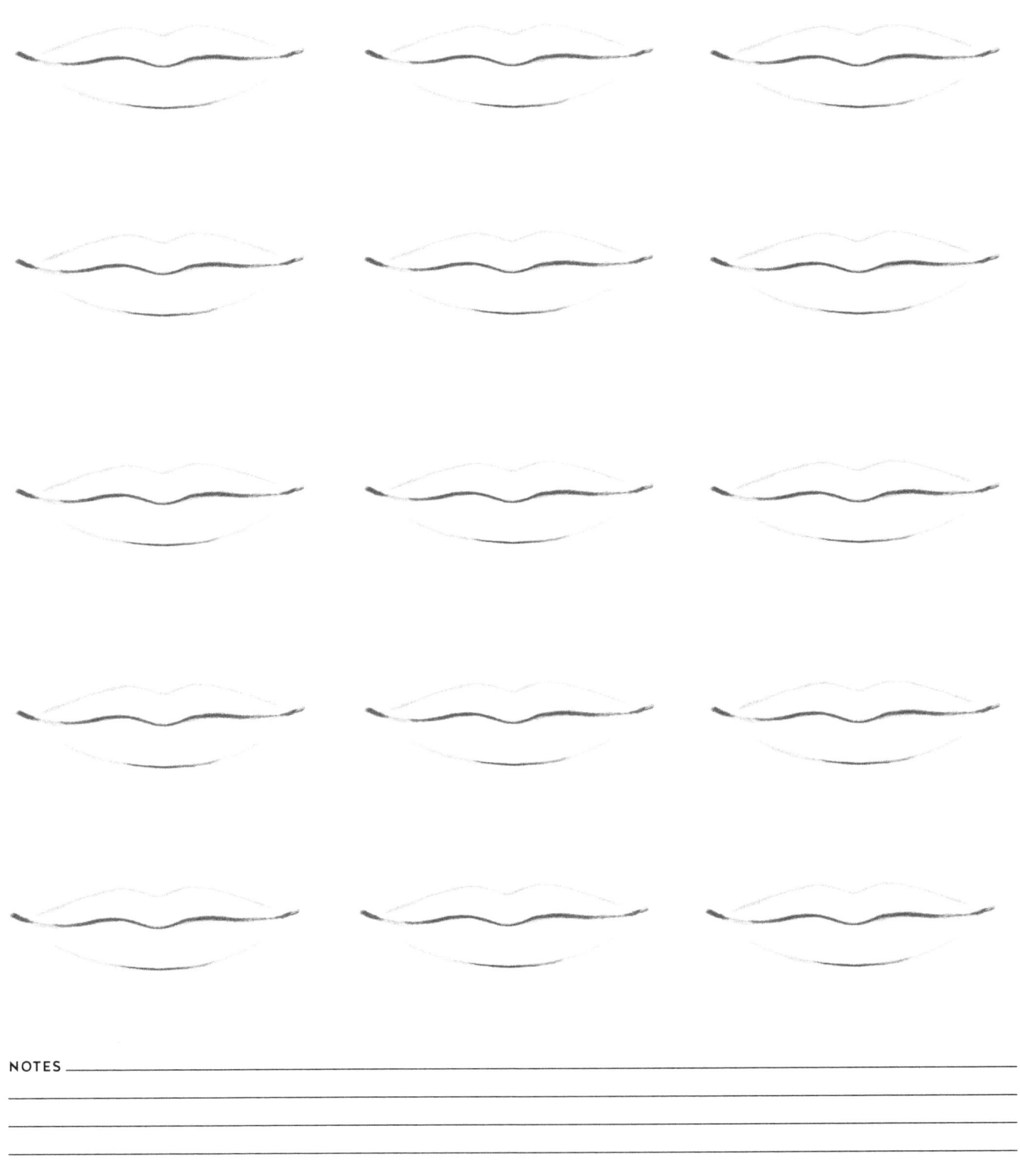

NOTES _____

_____

_____

_____

_____

LIP PRACTICE CHARTS

Use templates to design looks and practice application techniques.

Full Lip Shape

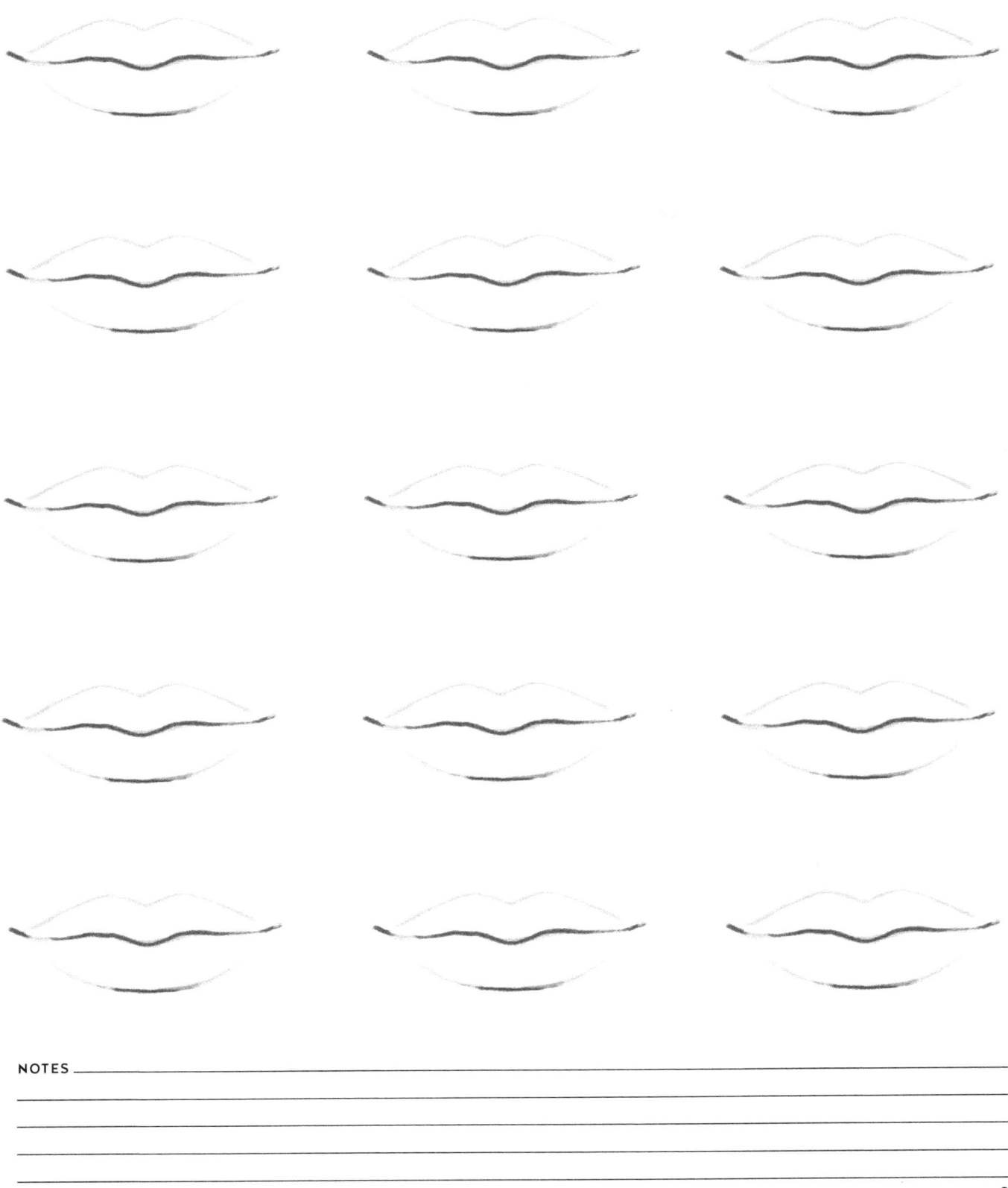

NOTES _____

_____

_____

_____

_____

LIP PRACTICE CHARTS

Use templates to design looks and practice application techniques.

Extra-full Lip Shape

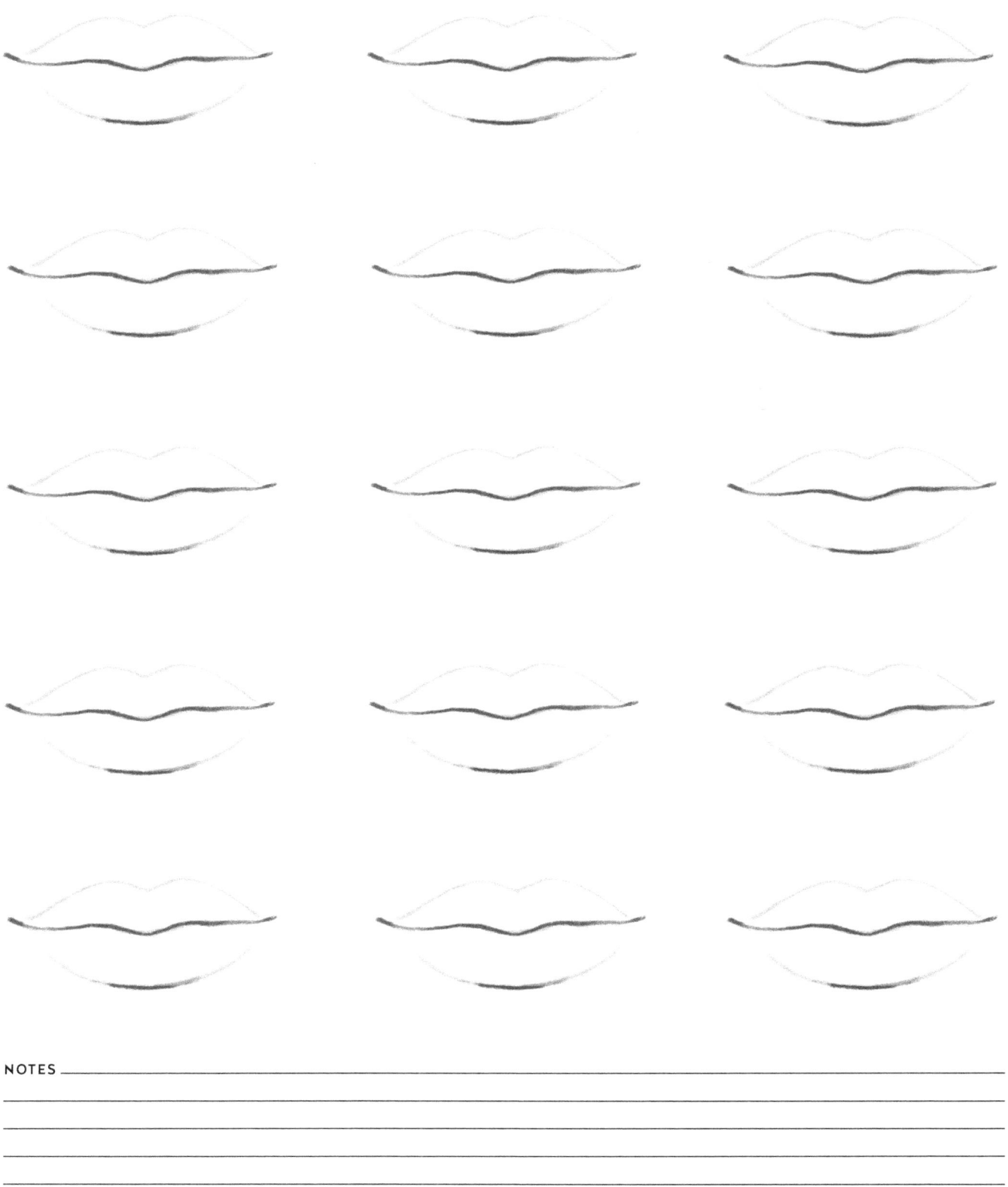

NOTES _____

_____

_____

_____

_____

makeup lip charts
Thin Shape

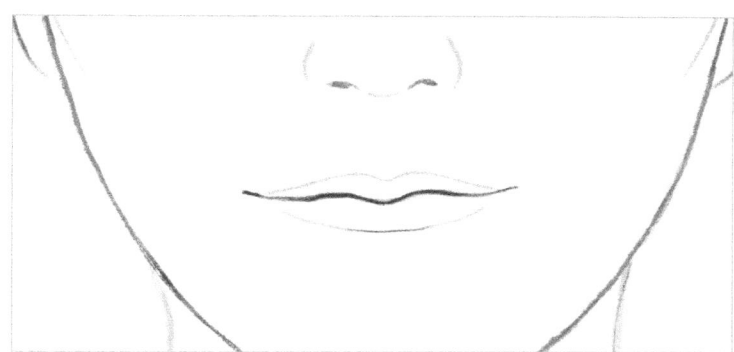

_____

_____

_____

_____

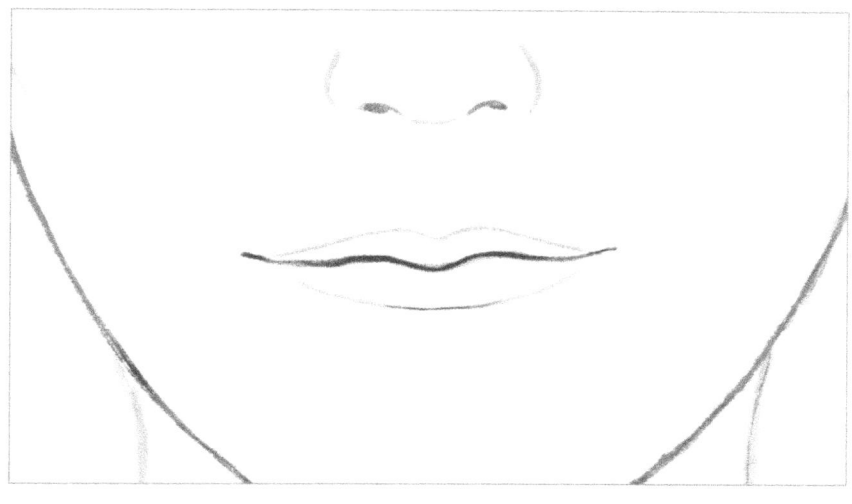

LOOK NAME_____

LIP SHAPE _Thin_____

LINER _____

COLOR _____

GLOSS _____

NOTES _____

_____

_____

_____

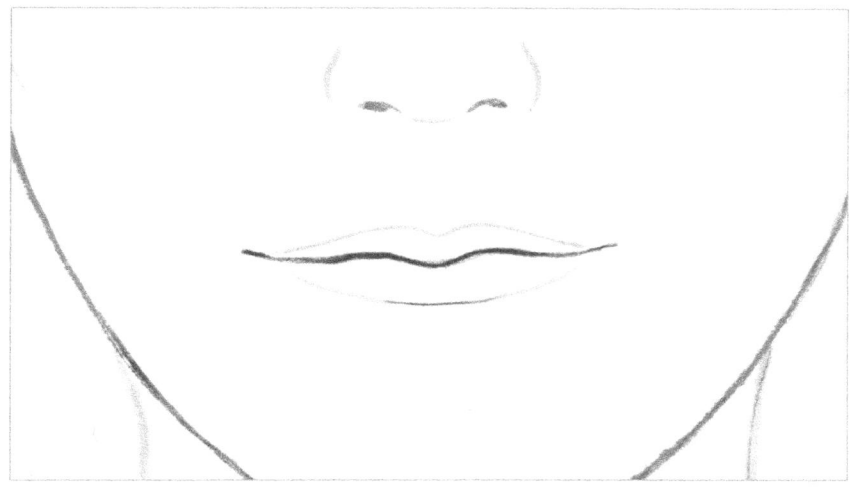

LOOK NAME_____

LIP SHAPE _Thin_____

LINER _____

COLOR _____

GLOSS _____

NOTES _____

_____

_____

_____

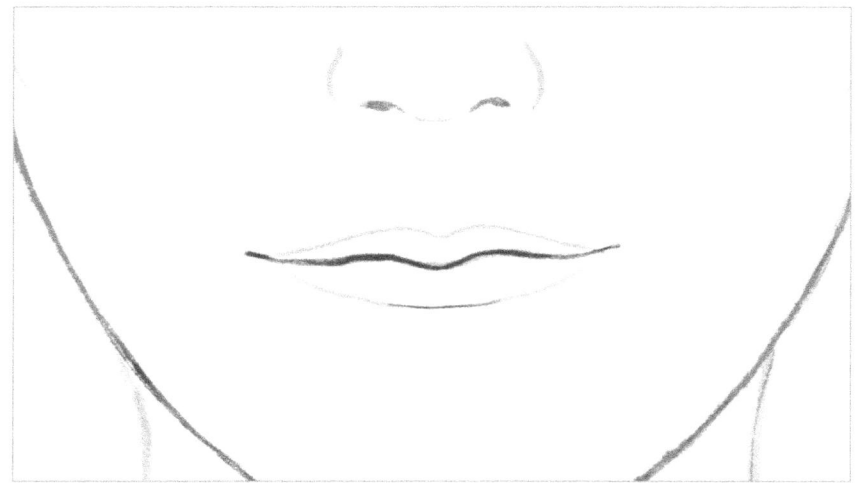

LOOK NAME_____

LIP SHAPE _Thin_____

LINER _____

COLOR _____

GLOSS _____

NOTES _____

_____

_____

_____

BRUSHES + TOOLS

_____

_____

_____

_____

NOTES

_____

_____

_____

_____

BRUSHES + TOOLS

_____

_____

_____

_____

NOTES

_____

_____

_____

_____

BRUSHES + TOOLS

_____

_____

_____

NOTES

_____

_____

_____

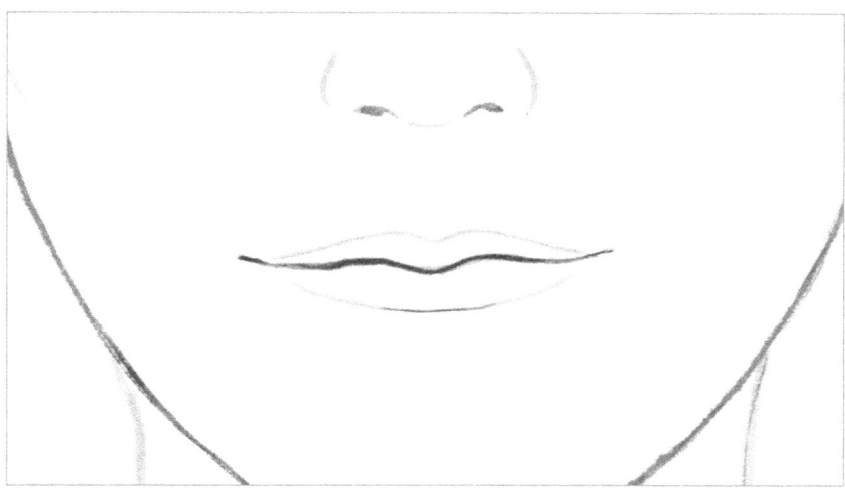

LOOK NAME_____

LIP SHAPE Thin_____

LINER _____

COLOR _____

GLOSS _____

NOTES_____

_____

_____

_____

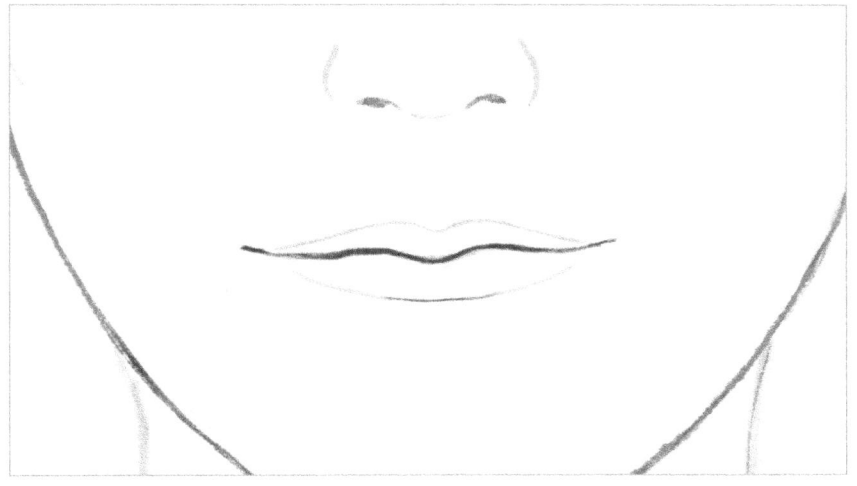

LOOK NAME_____

LIP SHAPE Thin_____

LINER _____

COLOR_____

GLOSS _____

NOTES_____

_____

_____

_____

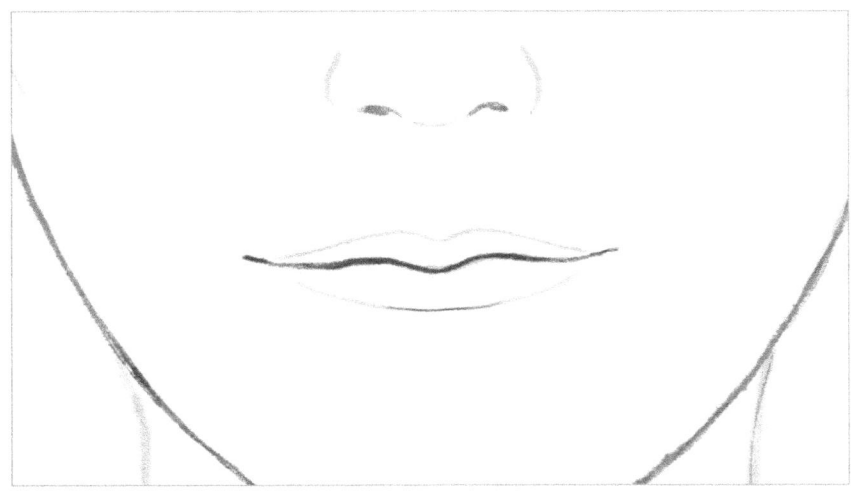

LOOK NAME_____

LIP SHAPE Thin_____

LINER _____

COLOR_____

GLOSS _____

NOTES_____

_____

_____

_____

BRUSHES + TOOLS

_____

_____

_____

_____

NOTES

_____

_____

_____

_____

. . . .

BRUSHES + TOOLS

_____

_____

_____

_____

NOTES

_____

_____

_____

_____

. . . .

BRUSHES + TOOLS

_____

_____

_____

_____

NOTES

_____

_____

_____

_____

makeup lip chart

LOOK NAME _____

LIP SHAPE Thin _____

LINER _____

COLOR _____

GLOSS _____

NOTES _____

CLIENT NAME _____

MAKEUP ARTIST _____

makeup lip chart

LOOK NAME _____

LIP SHAPE Thin _____

LINER _____

COLOR _____

GLOSS _____

NOTES _____

CLIENT NAME _____

MAKEUP ARTIST _____

BRUSHES + TOOLS

_____

_____

_____

· ·

NOTES

_____

_____

_____

BRUSHES + TOOLS

_____

_____

_____

NOTES

_____

_____

_____

makeup lip chart

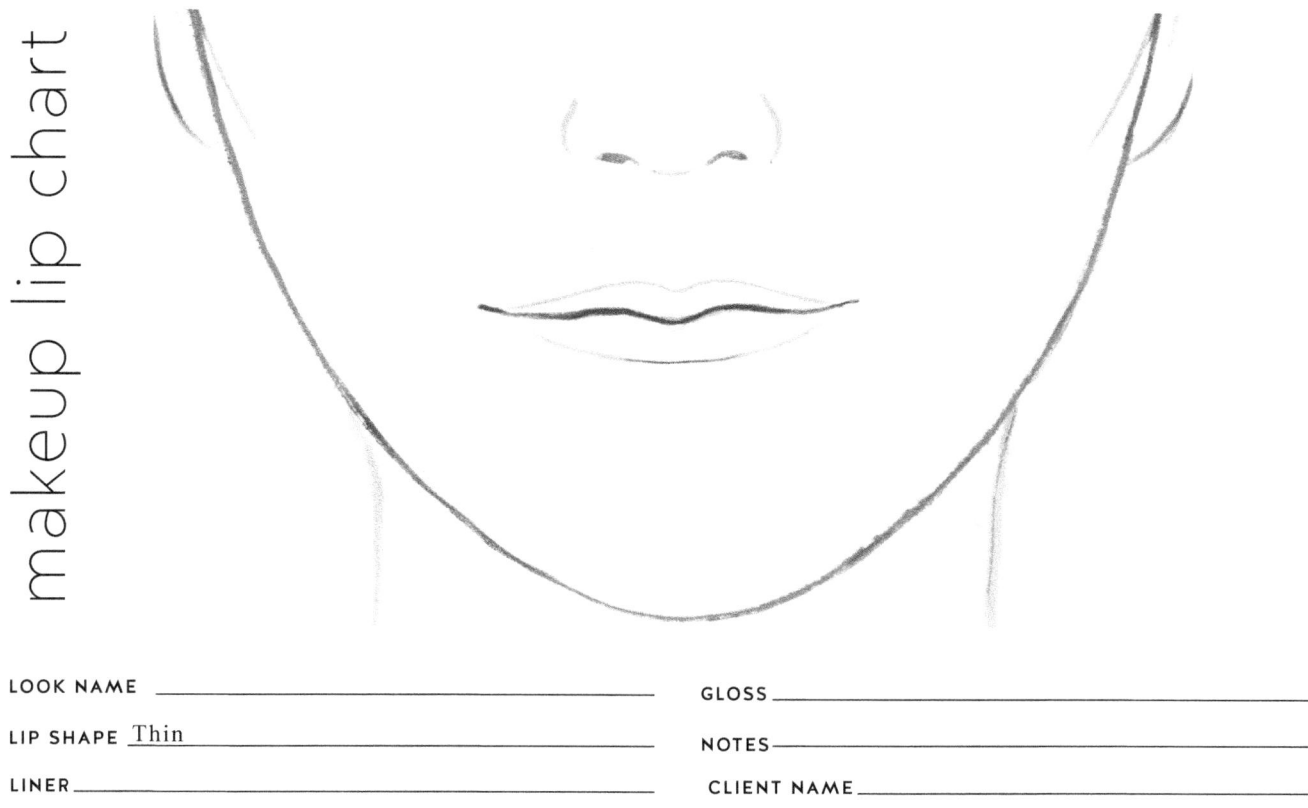

LOOK NAME _____

LIP SHAPE Thin _____

LINER _____

COLOR _____

GLOSS _____

NOTES _____

CLIENT NAME _____

MAKEUP ARTIST _____

....

makeup lip chart

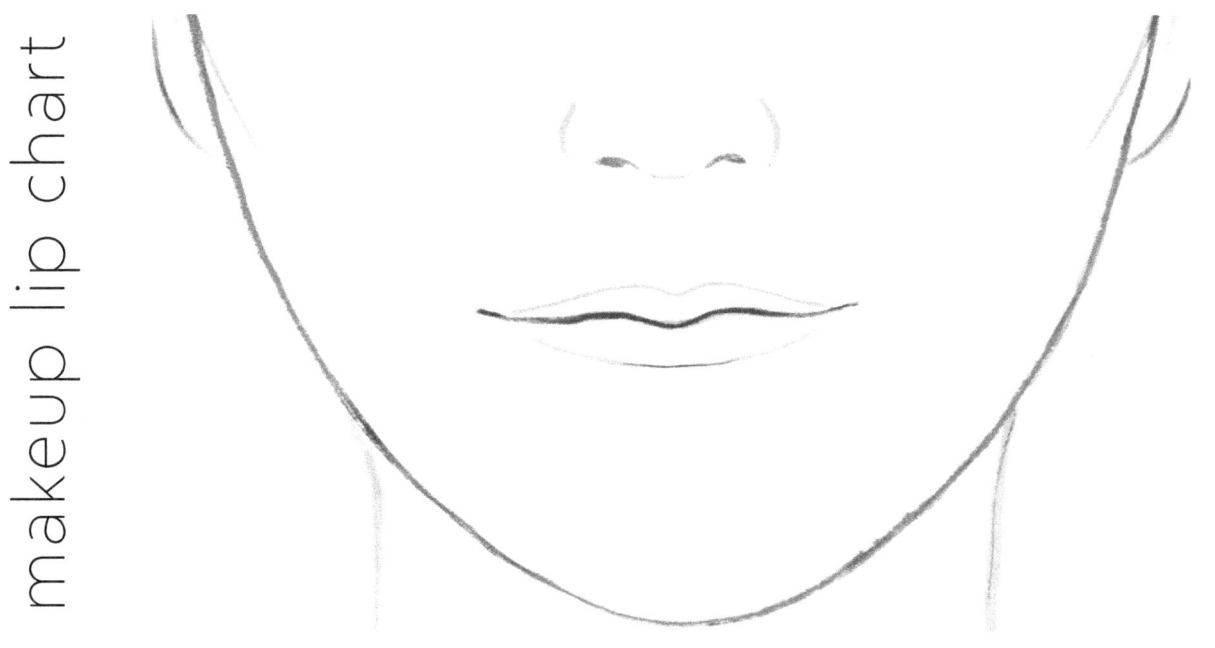

LOOK NAME _____

LIP SHAPE Thin _____

LINER _____

COLOR _____

GLOSS _____

NOTES _____

CLIENT NAME _____

MAKEUP ARTIST _____

BRUSHES + TOOLS

_____

_____

_____

· ·

NOTES

_____

_____

_____

BRUSHES + TOOLS

_____

_____

_____

NOTES

_____

_____

_____

makeup lip chart

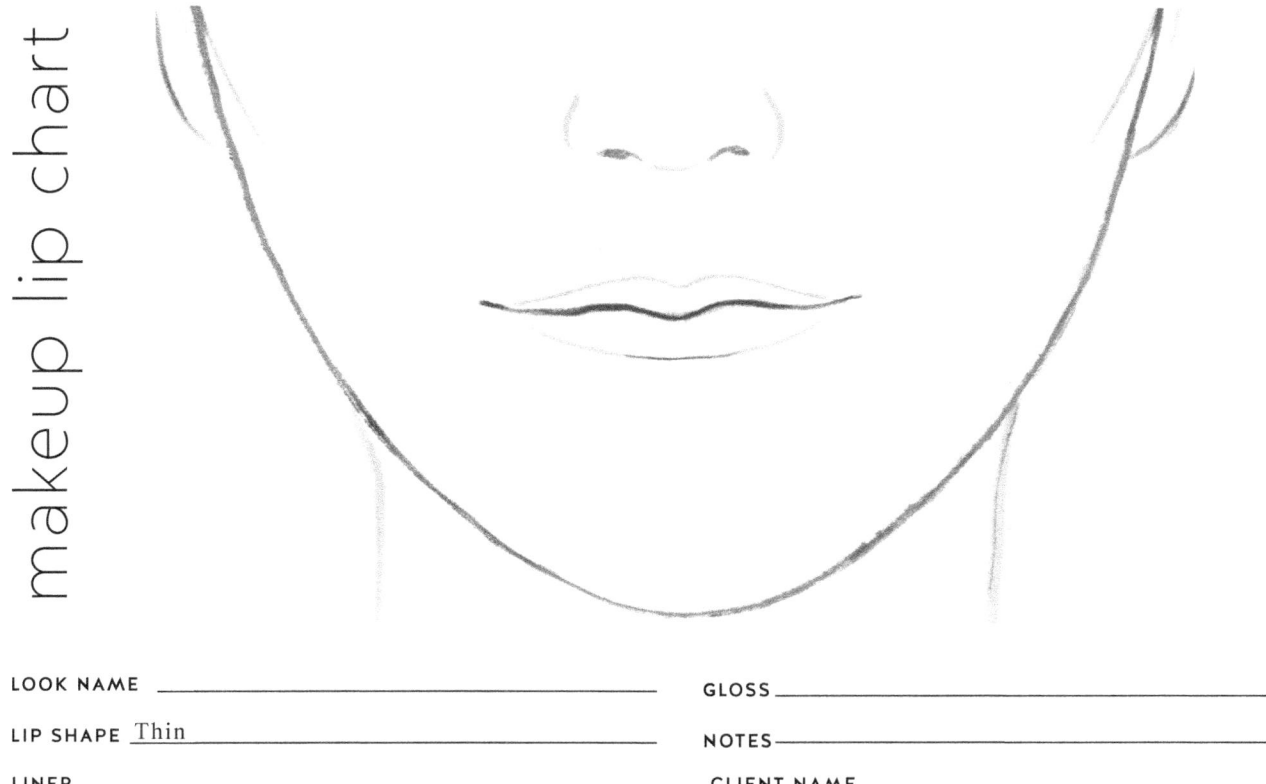

LOOK NAME _____

LIP SHAPE <u>Thin</u>_____

LINER _____

COLOR _____

GLOSS _____

NOTES _____

CLIENT NAME _____

MAKEUP ARTIST _____

makeup lip chart

LOOK NAME _____

LIP SHAPE <u>Thin</u>_____

LINER _____

COLOR _____

GLOSS _____

NOTES _____

CLIENT NAME _____

MAKEUP ARTIST _____

BRUSHES + TOOLS

NOTES

_____

_____

_____

_____

_____

_____

· ·

BRUSHES + TOOLS

NOTES

_____

_____

_____

_____

_____

_____

makeup lip charts
Thin-upper Shape

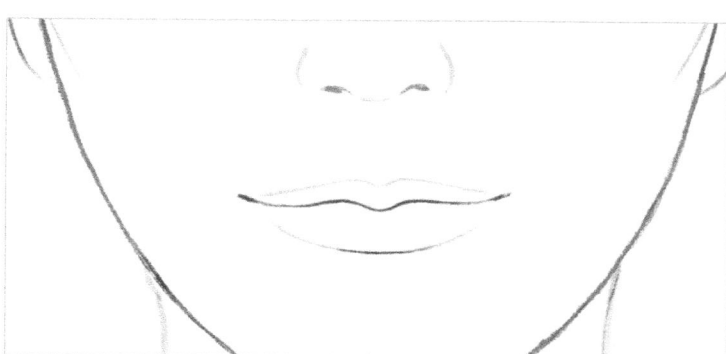

_____

_____

_____

_____

makeup lip charts

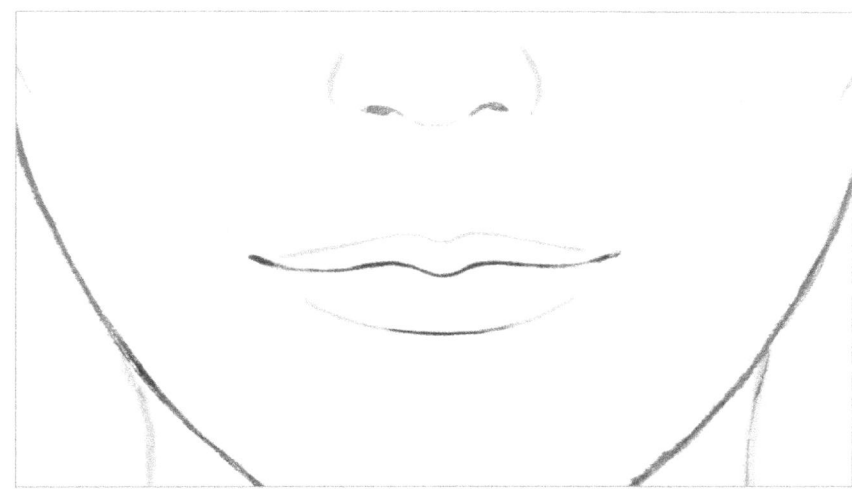

LOOK NAME_____

LIP SHAPE _Thin-upper_____

LINER _____

COLOR _____

GLOSS _____

NOTES _____

_____

_____

_____

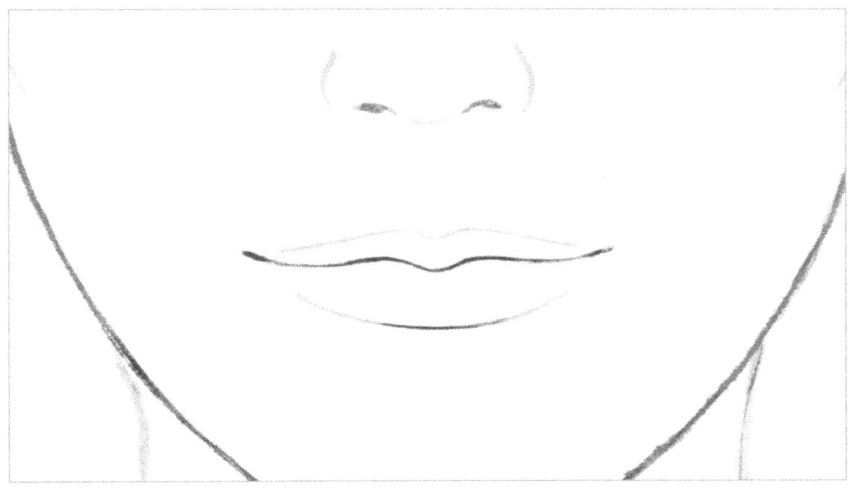

LOOK NAME_____

LIP SHAPE _Thin-upper_____

LINER _____

COLOR _____

GLOSS _____

NOTES _____

_____

_____

_____

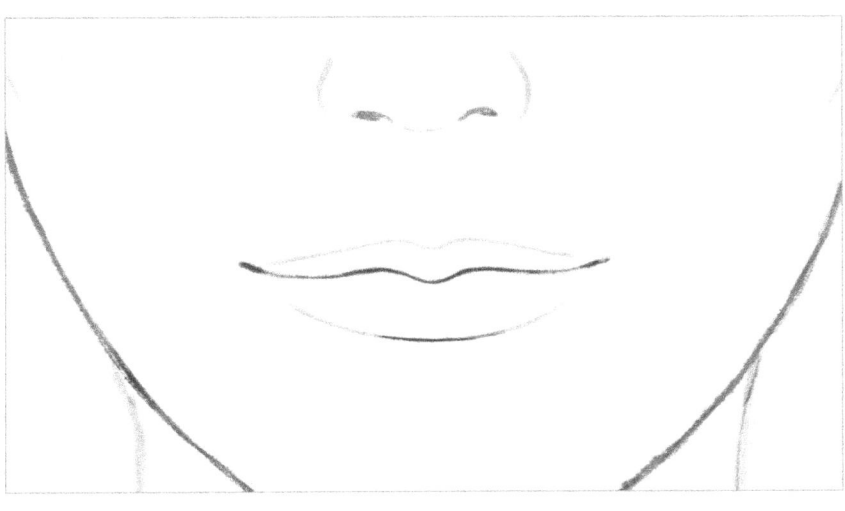

LOOK NAME_____

LIP SHAPE _Thin-upper_____

LINER _____

COLOR _____

GLOSS _____

NOTES _____

_____

_____

_____

BRUSHES + TOOLS

NOTES

_____

_____

_____

_____

BRUSHES + TOOLS

NOTES

_____

_____

_____

_____

BRUSHES + TOOLS

NOTES

_____

_____

_____

_____

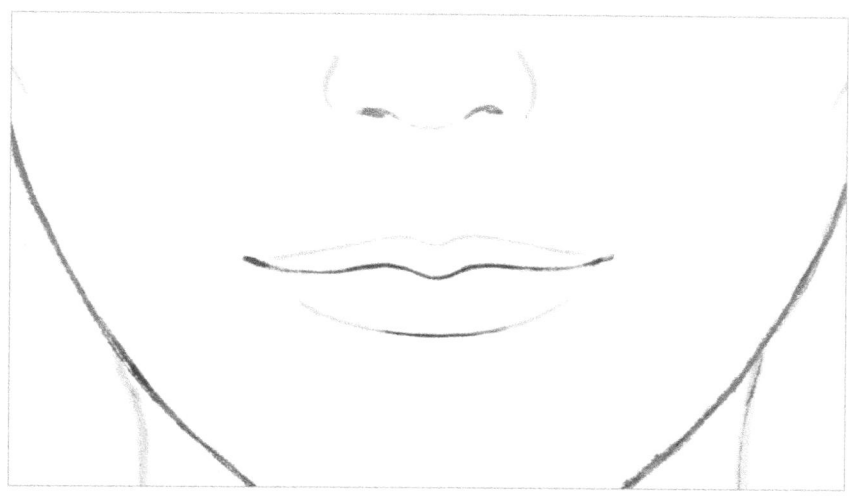

LOOK NAME _____

LIP SHAPE _Thin-upper_____

LINER _____

COLOR _____

GLOSS _____

NOTES _____

_____

_____

_____

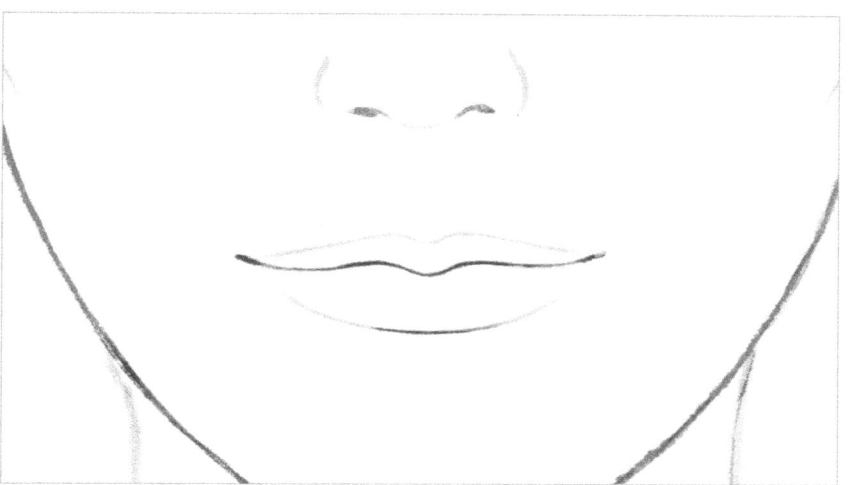

LOOK NAME _____

LIP SHAPE _Thin-upper_____

LINER _____

COLOR _____

GLOSS _____

NOTES _____

_____

_____

_____

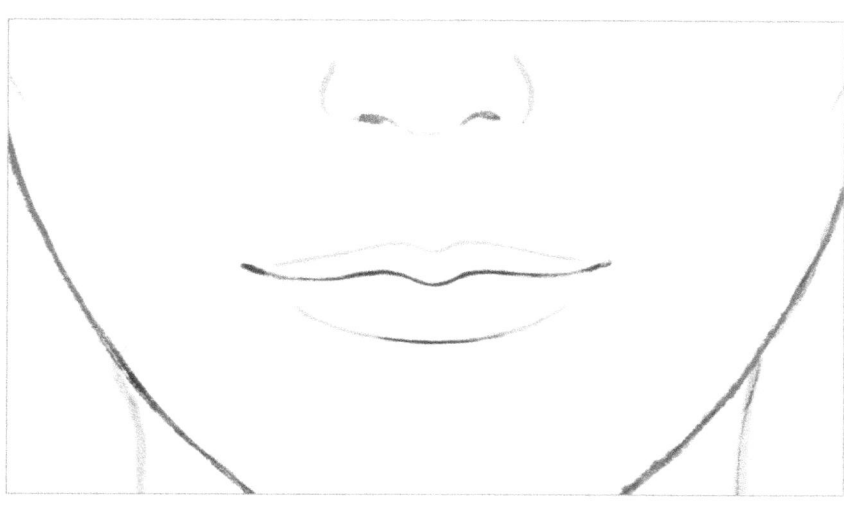

LOOK NAME _____

LIP SHAPE _Thin-upper_____

LINER _____

COLOR _____

GLOSS _____

NOTES _____

_____

_____

_____

BRUSHES + TOOLS

_____

_____

_____

_____

NOTES

_____

_____

_____

_____

....

BRUSHES + TOOLS

_____

_____

_____

_____

NOTES

_____

_____

_____

_____

....

BRUSHES + TOOLS

_____

_____

_____

_____

NOTES

_____

_____

_____

_____

makeup lip chart

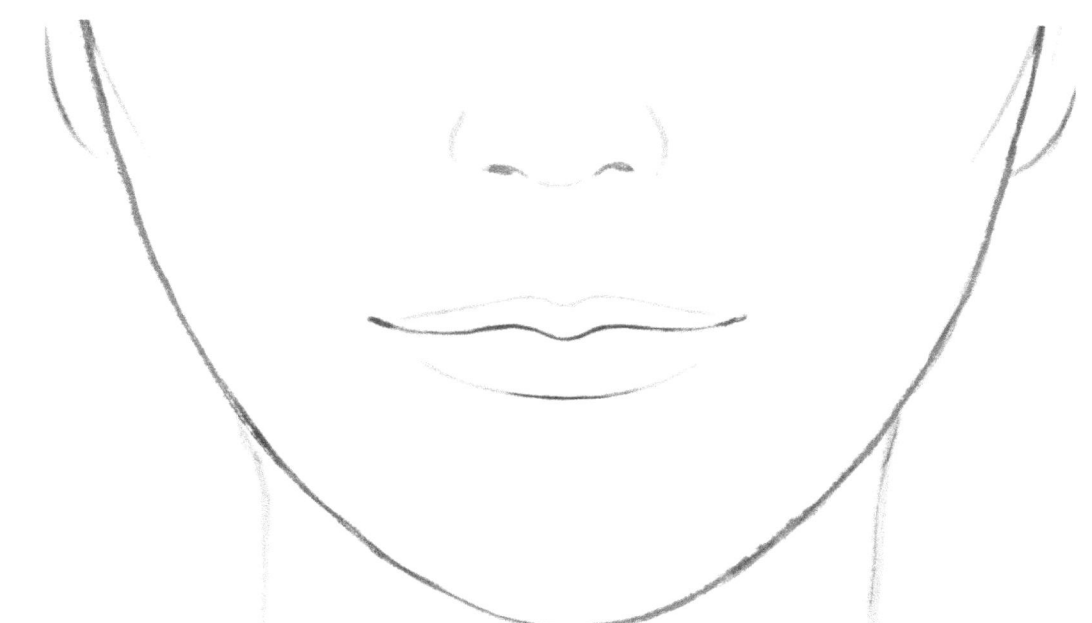

LOOK NAME _____

LIP SHAPE <u>Thin-upper</u> _____

LINER _____

COLOR _____

GLOSS _____

NOTES _____

CLIENT NAME _____

MAKEUP ARTIST _____

makeup lip chart

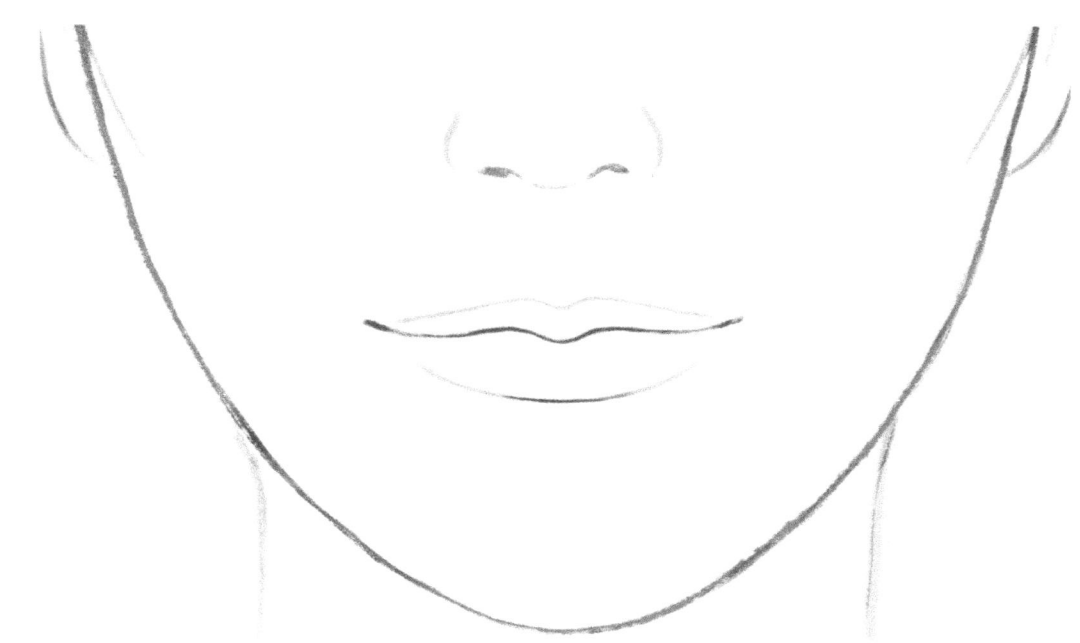

LOOK NAME _____

LIP SHAPE <u>Thin-upper</u> _____

LINER _____

COLOR _____

GLOSS _____

NOTES _____

CLIENT NAME _____

MAKEUP ARTIST _____

BRUSHES + TOOLS

_____

_____

_____

· ·

NOTES

_____

_____

_____

BRUSHES + TOOLS

_____

_____

_____

NOTES

_____

_____

_____

makeup lip chart

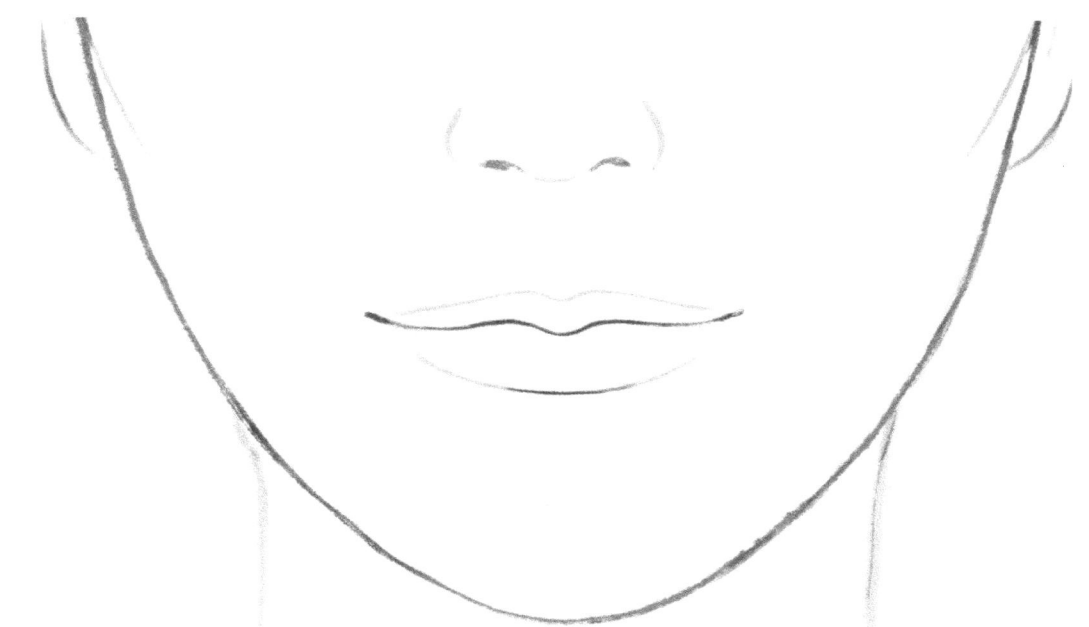

LOOK NAME _____

LIP SHAPE <u>Thin-upper</u> _____

LINER _____

COLOR _____

GLOSS _____

NOTES _____

CLIENT NAME _____

MAKEUP ARTIST _____

makeup lip chart

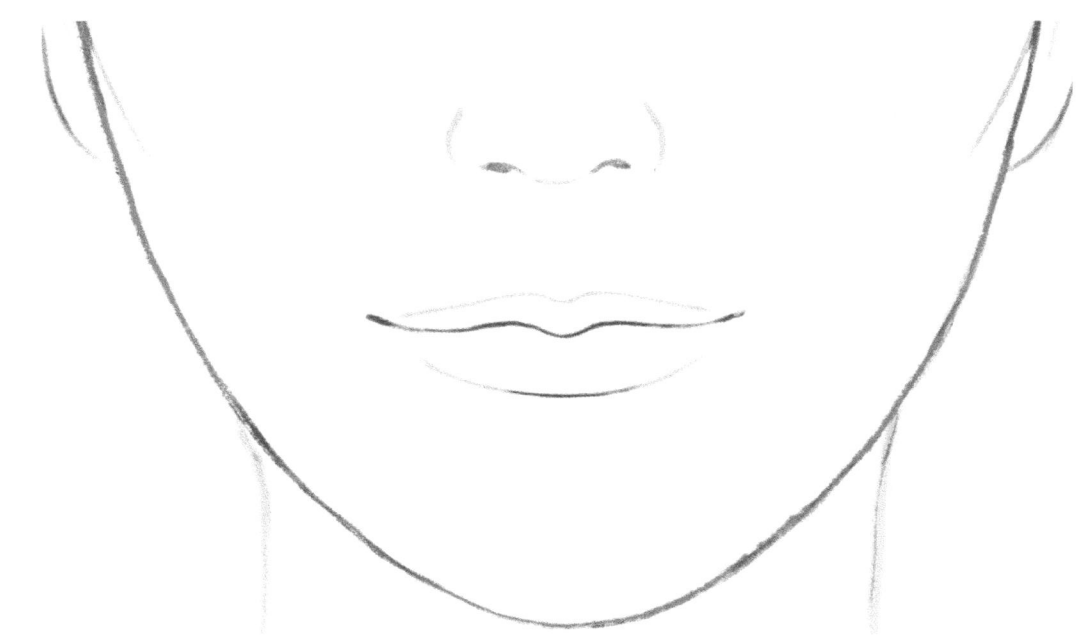

LOOK NAME _____

LIP SHAPE <u>Thin-upper</u> _____

LINER _____

COLOR _____

GLOSS _____

NOTES _____

CLIENT NAME _____

MAKEUP ARTIST _____

BRUSHES + TOOLS

_____

_____

_____

....

NOTES

_____

_____

_____

BRUSHES + TOOLS

_____

_____

_____

NOTES

_____

_____

_____

makeup lip chart

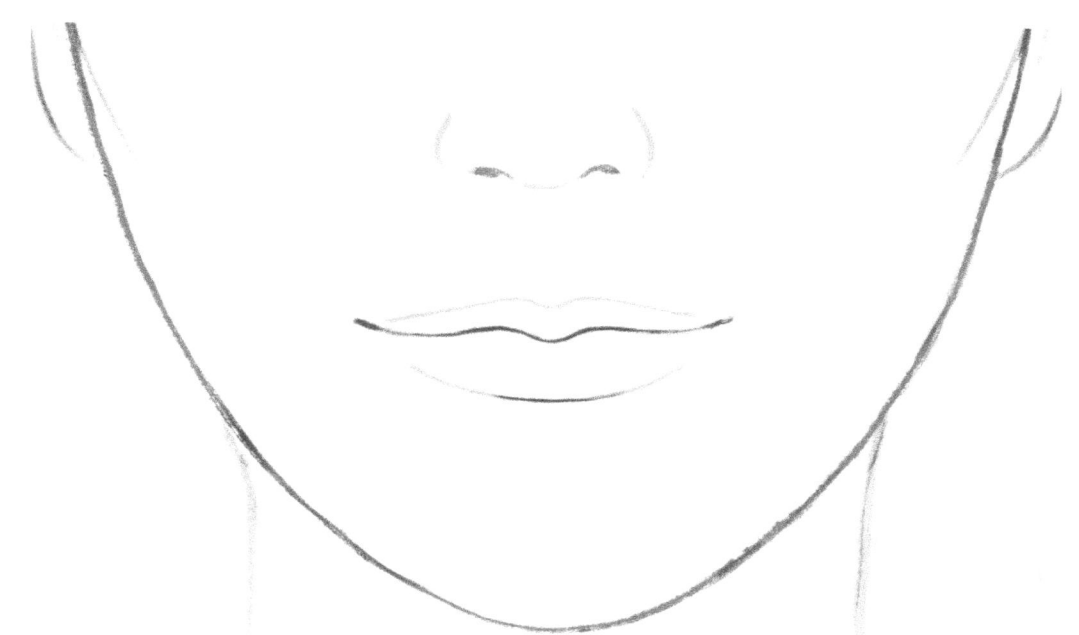

LOOK NAME _____

LIP SHAPE <u>Thin-upper</u> _____

LINER _____

COLOR _____

GLOSS _____

NOTES _____

CLIENT NAME _____

MAKEUP ARTIST _____

makeup lip chart

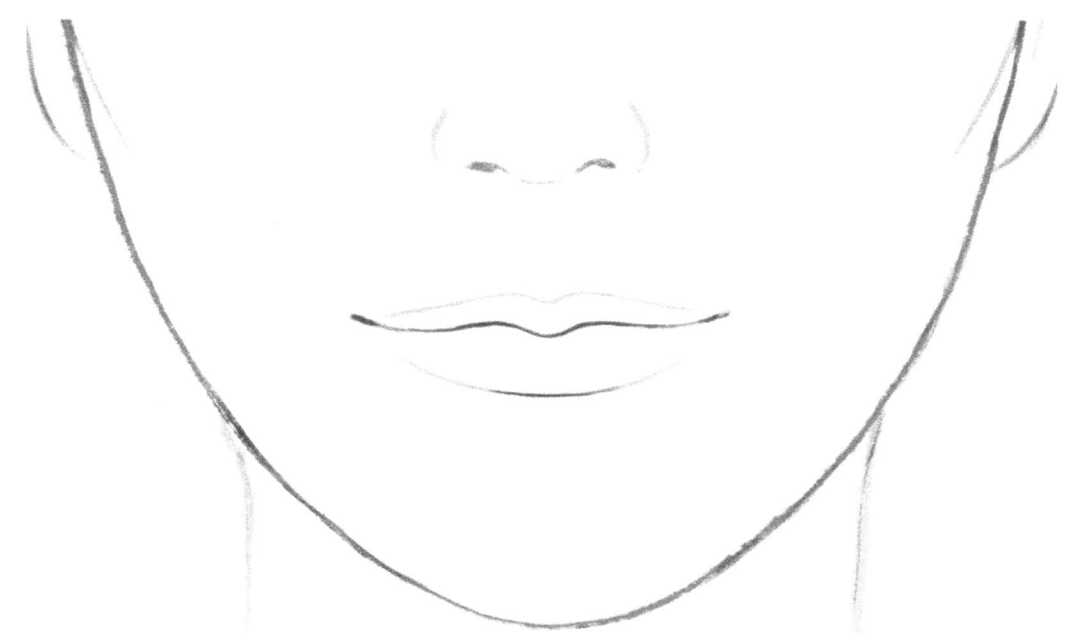

LOOK NAME _____

LIP SHAPE <u>Thin-upper</u> _____

LINER _____

COLOR _____

GLOSS _____

NOTES _____

CLIENT NAME _____

MAKEUP ARTIST _____

BRUSHES + TOOLS

NOTES

_____

_____

_____

BRUSHES + TOOLS

NOTES

_____

_____

_____

makeup lip charts
Thin-lower Shape

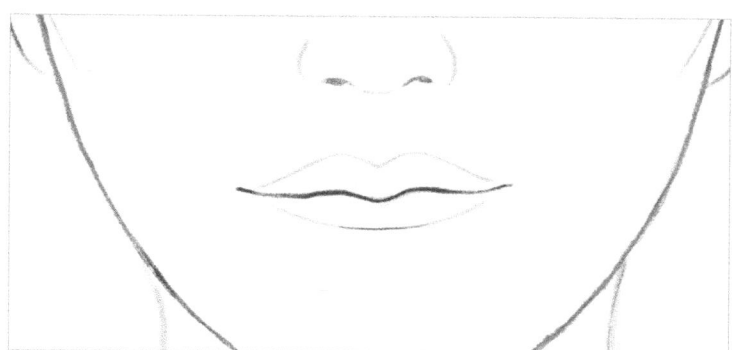

_____

_____

_____

_____

_____

_____

_____

_____

_____

_____

_____

_____

_____

_____

_____

_____

_____

_____

_____

_____

_____

_____

_____

_____

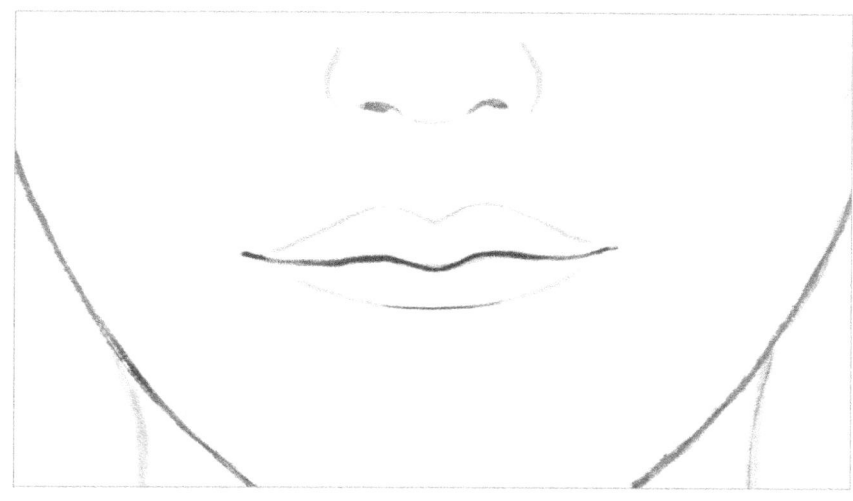

LOOK NAME _____

LIP SHAPE _Thin-lower_____

LINER _____

COLOR _____

GLOSS _____

NOTES _____

_____

_____

_____

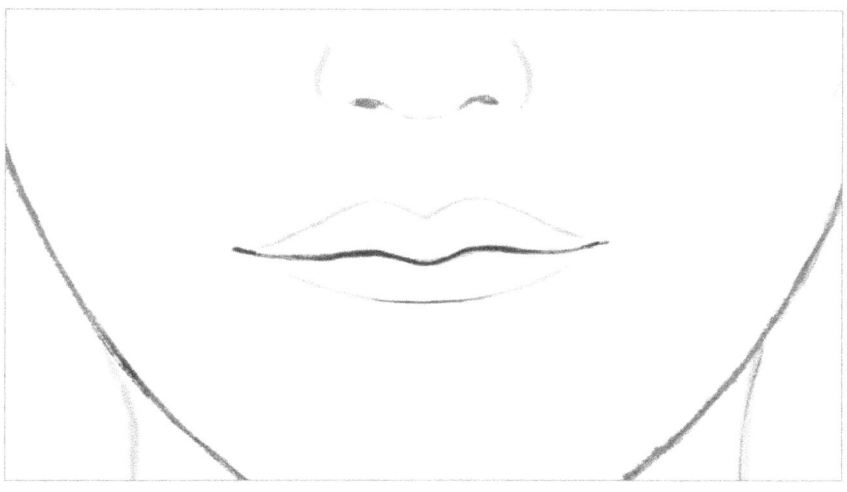

LOOK NAME _____

LIP SHAPE _Thin-lower_____

LINER _____

COLOR _____

GLOSS _____

NOTES _____

_____

_____

_____

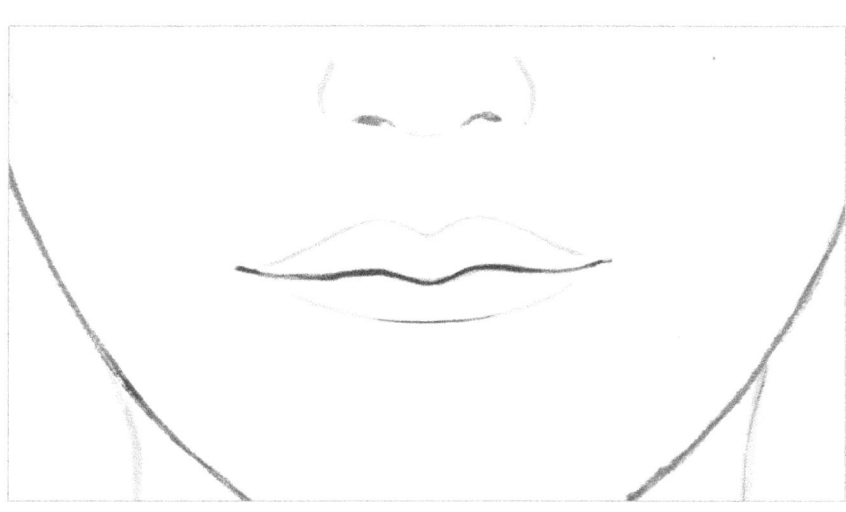

LOOK NAME _____

LIP SHAPE _Thin-lower_____

LINER _____

COLOR _____

GLOSS _____

NOTES _____

_____

_____

_____

BRUSHES + TOOLS

_____

_____

_____

_____

NOTES

_____

_____

_____

_____

BRUSHES + TOOLS

_____

_____

_____

_____

NOTES

_____

_____

_____

_____

BRUSHES + TOOLS

_____

_____

_____

_____

NOTES

_____

_____

_____

_____

makeup lip charts

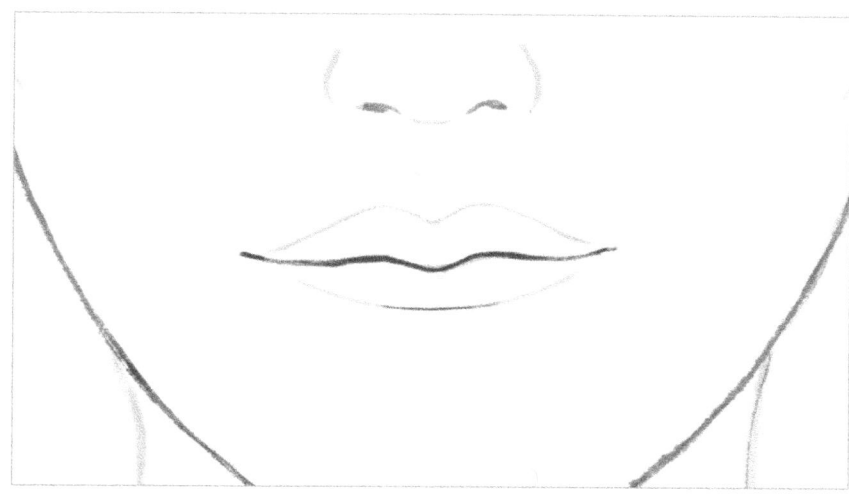

LOOK NAME_____

LIP SHAPE Thin-lower_____

LINER_____

COLOR_____

GLOSS_____

NOTES_____

_____

_____

_____

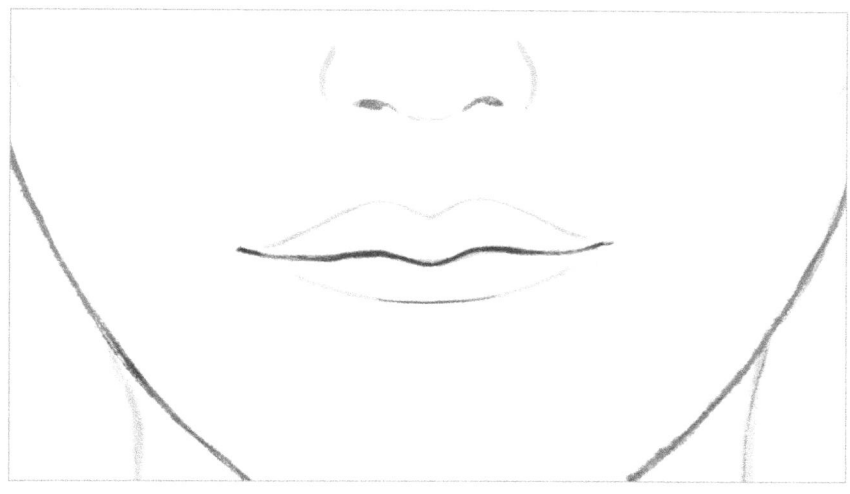

LOOK NAME_____

LIP SHAPE Thin-lower_____

LINER_____

COLOR_____

GLOSS_____

NOTES_____

_____

_____

_____

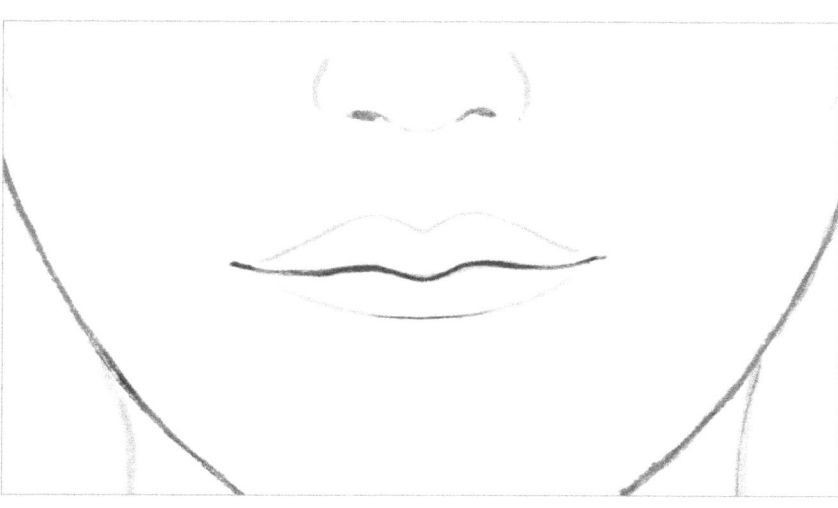

LOOK NAME_____

LIP SHAPE Thin-lower_____

LINER_____

COLOR_____

GLOSS_____

NOTES_____

_____

_____

_____

BRUSHES + TOOLS

_____

_____

_____

_____

NOTES

_____

_____

_____

_____

BRUSHES + TOOLS

_____

_____

_____

_____

NOTES

_____

_____

_____

_____

BRUSHES + TOOLS

_____

_____

_____

_____

NOTES

_____

_____

_____

_____

makeup lip chart

LOOK NAME _____

LIP SHAPE <u>Thin-lower</u>_____

LINER _____

COLOR _____

GLOSS _____

NOTES _____

CLIENT NAME _____

MAKEUP ARTIST _____

....

makeup lip chart

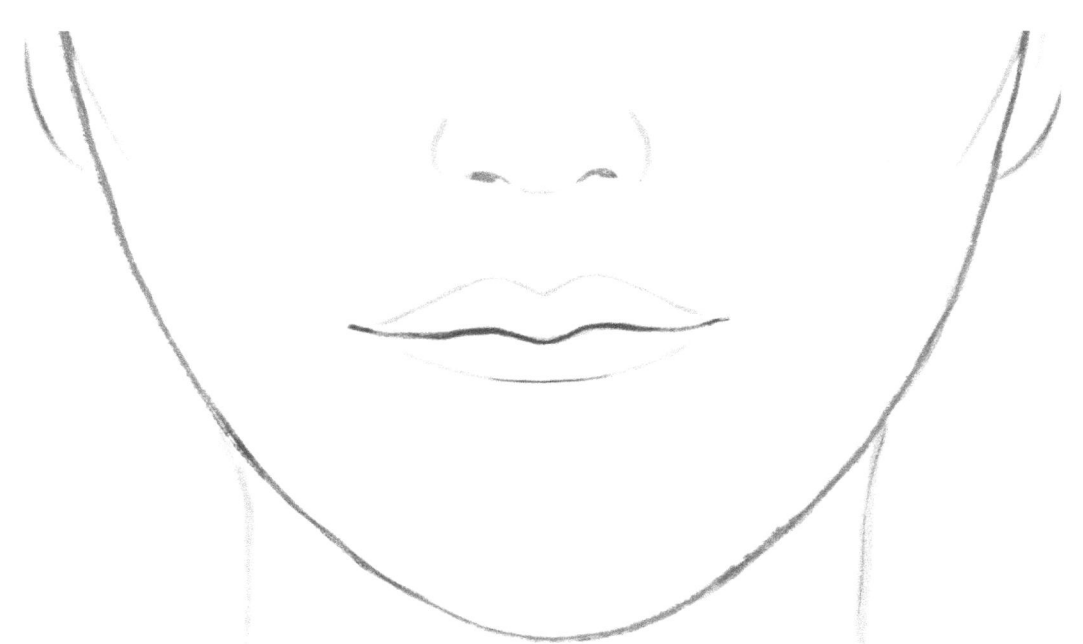

LOOK NAME _____

LIP SHAPE <u>Thin-lower</u>_____

LINER _____

COLOR _____

GLOSS _____

NOTES _____

CLIENT NAME _____

MAKEUP ARTIST _____

BRUSHES + TOOLS

_____

_____

_____

NOTES

_____

_____

_____

BRUSHES + TOOLS

_____

_____

_____

NOTES

_____

_____

_____

makeup lip chart

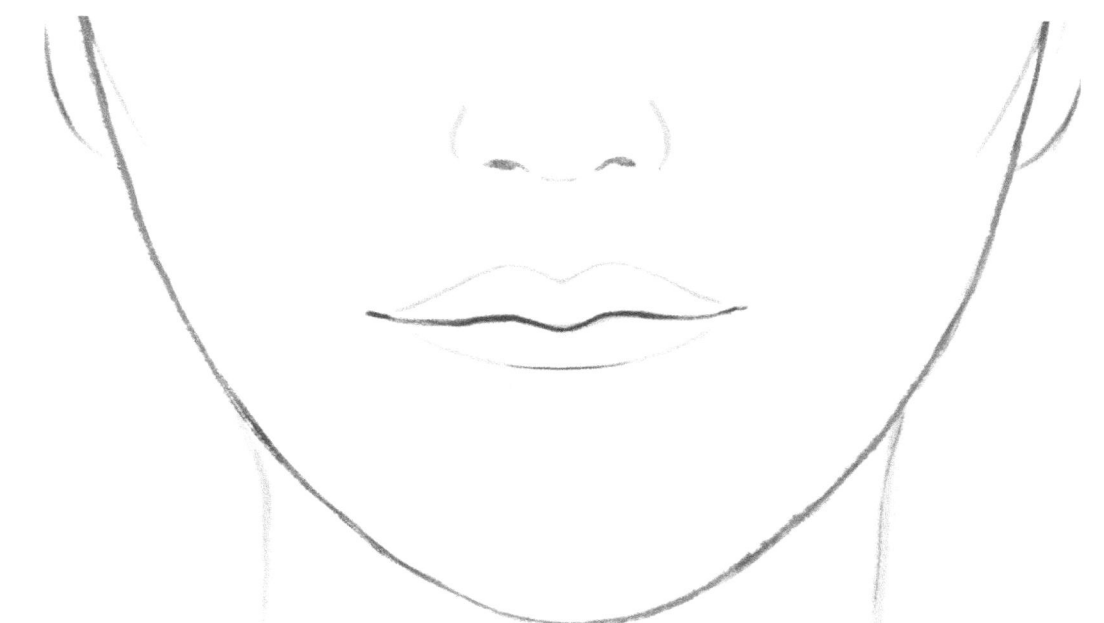

LOOK NAME _____

LIP SHAPE <u>Thin-lower</u>_____

LINER _____

COLOR _____

GLOSS _____

NOTES _____

  CLIENT NAME _____

MAKEUP ARTIST _____

···

makeup lip chart

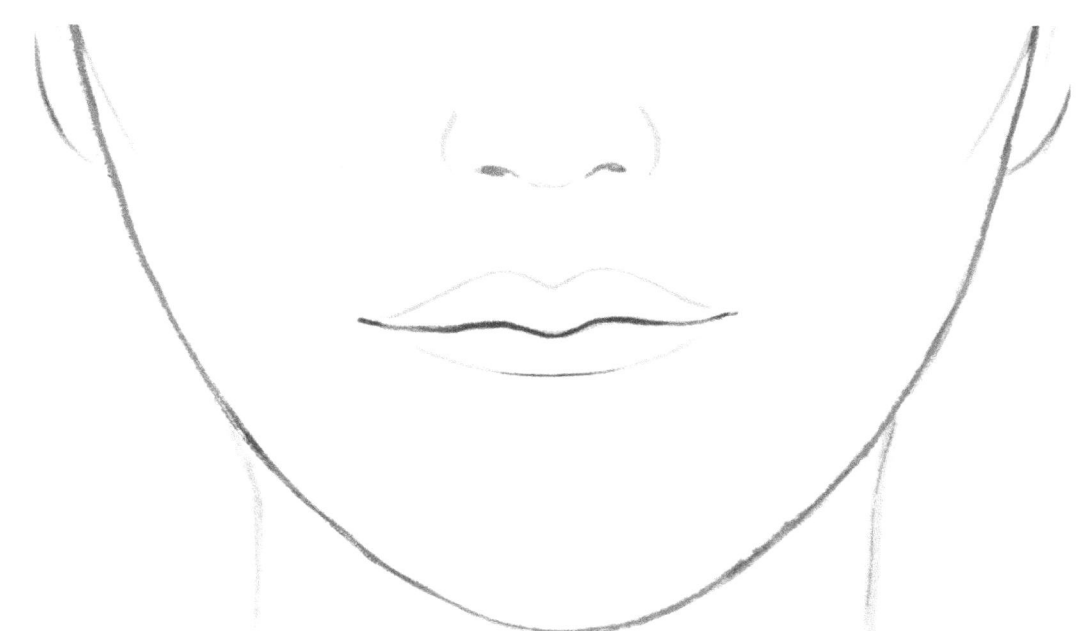

LOOK NAME _____

LIP SHAPE <u>Thin-lower</u>_____

LINER _____

COLOR _____

GLOSS _____

NOTES _____

  CLIENT NAME _____

MAKEUP ARTIST _____

BRUSHES + TOOLS

_____

_____

_____

· ·

NOTES

_____

_____

_____

BRUSHES + TOOLS

_____

_____

_____

NOTES

_____

_____

_____

makeup lip chart

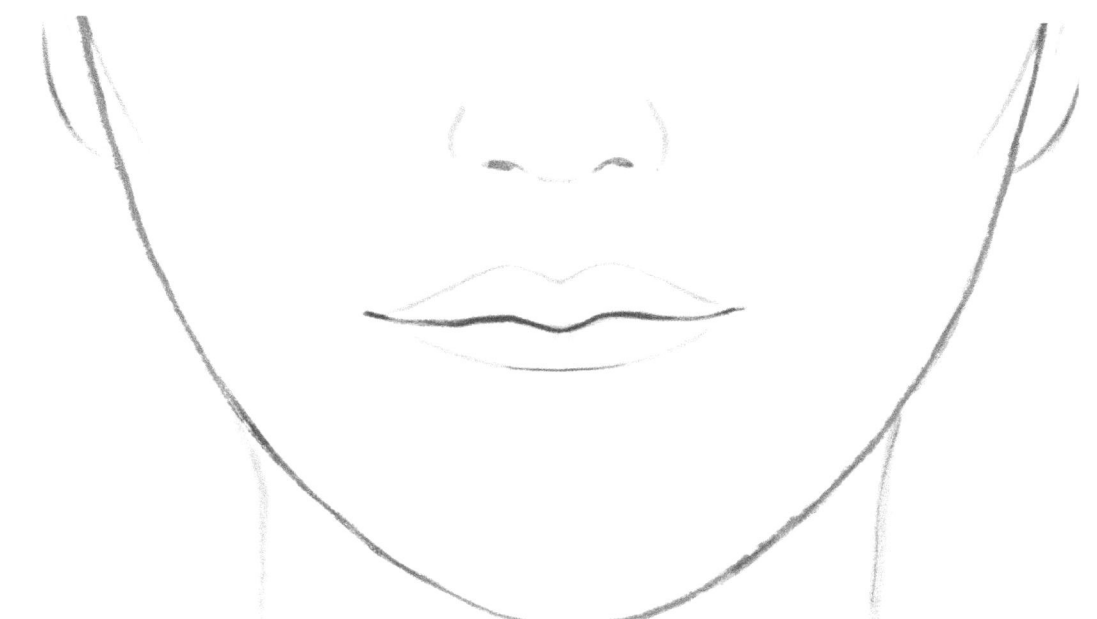

LOOK NAME _____

LIP SHAPE <u>Thin-lower</u> _____

LINER _____

COLOR _____

GLOSS _____

NOTES _____

CLIENT NAME _____

MAKEUP ARTIST _____

makeup lip chart

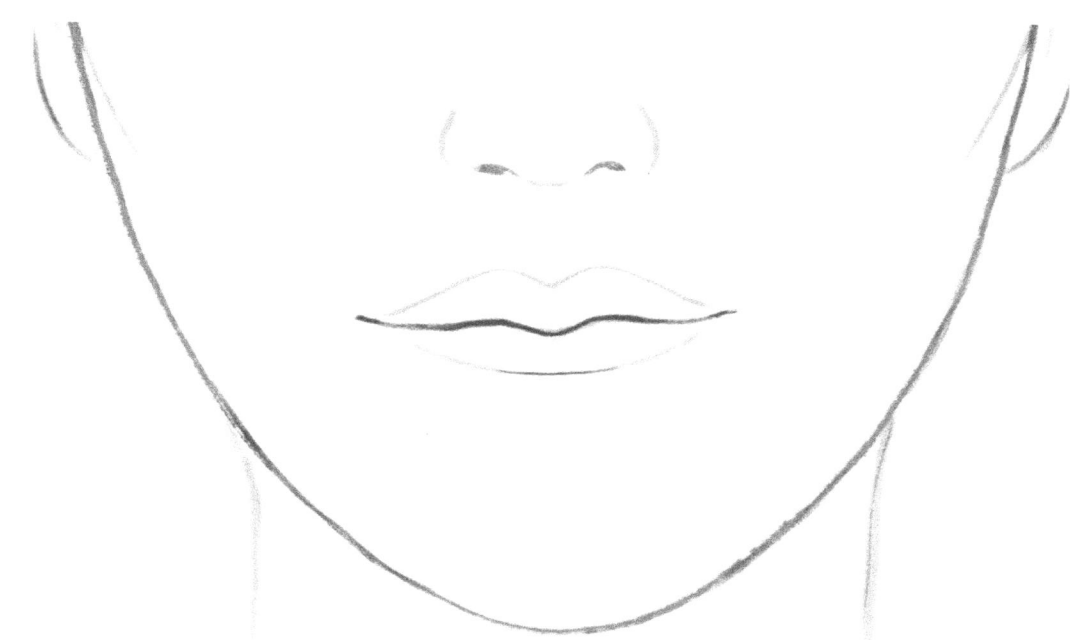

LOOK NAME _____

LIP SHAPE <u>Thin-lower</u> _____

LINER _____

COLOR _____

GLOSS _____

NOTES _____

CLIENT NAME _____

MAKEUP ARTIST _____

BRUSHES + TOOLS

_____

_____

_____

· ·

NOTES

_____

_____

_____

BRUSHES + TOOLS

_____

_____

_____

NOTES

_____

_____

_____

makeup lip charts
Medium Shape

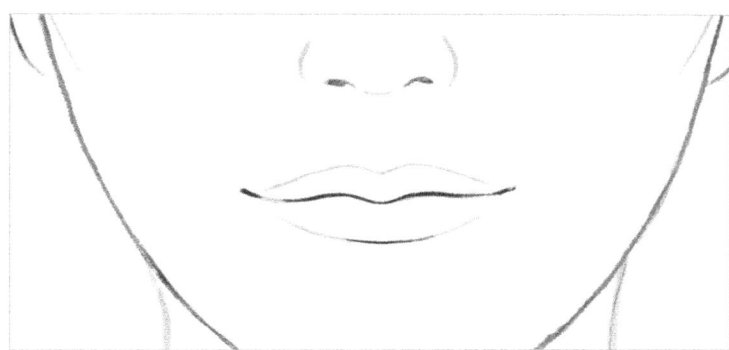

makeup lip charts

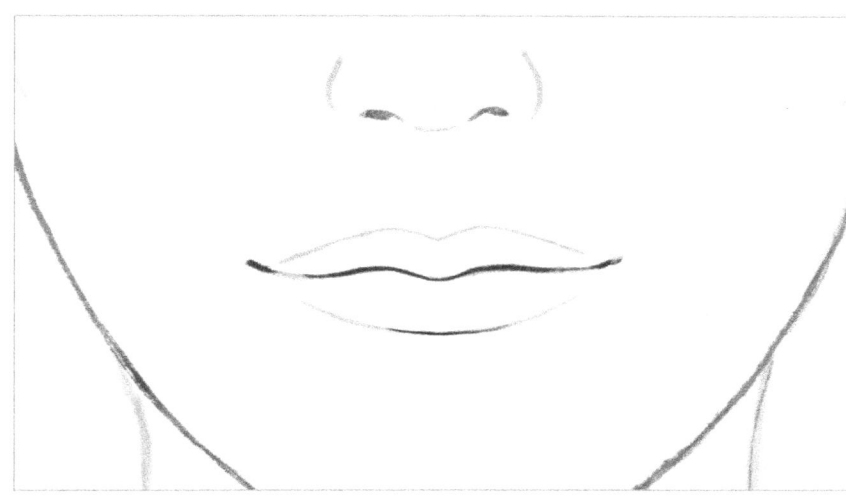

LOOK NAME_____

LIP SHAPE _Medium_____

LINER_____

COLOR_____

GLOSS_____

NOTES_____

_____

_____

_____

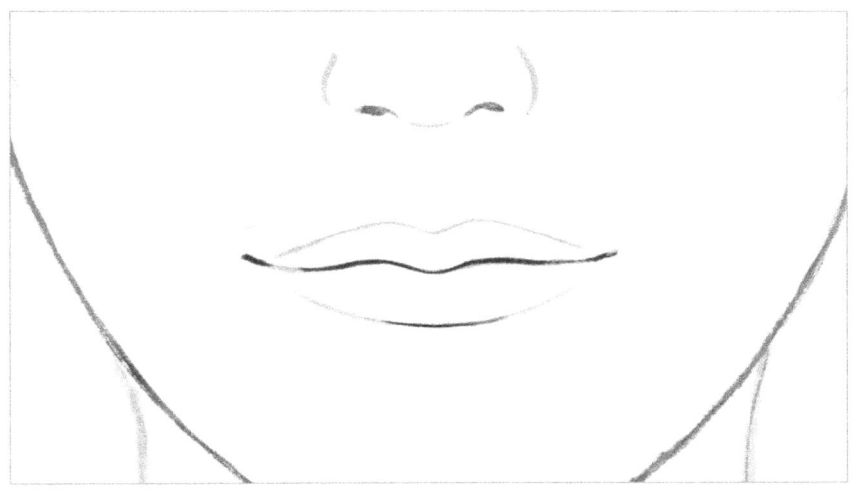

LOOK NAME_____

LIP SHAPE _Medium_____

LINER_____

COLOR_____

GLOSS_____

NOTES_____

_____

_____

_____

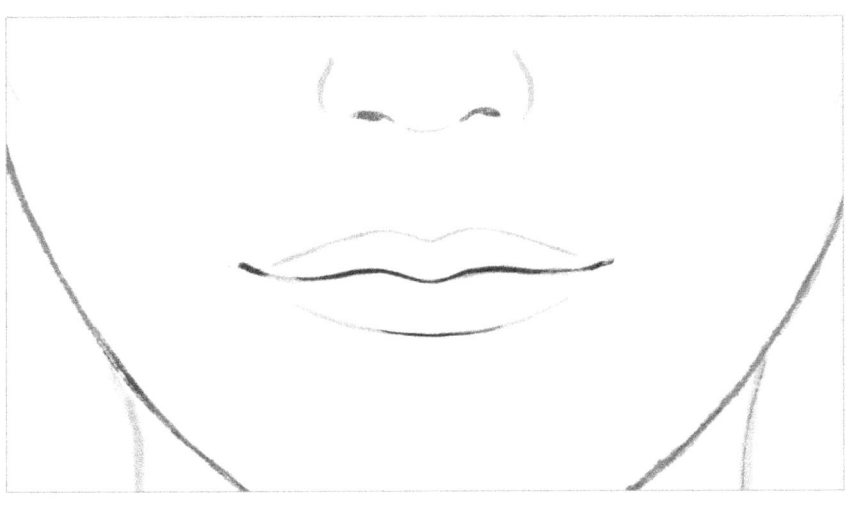

LOOK NAME_____

LIP SHAPE _Medium_____

LINER_____

COLOR_____

GLOSS_____

NOTES_____

_____

_____

_____

BRUSHES + TOOLS

_____

_____

_____

_____

NOTES

_____

_____

_____

_____

BRUSHES + TOOLS

_____

_____

_____

_____

NOTES

_____

_____

_____

_____

BRUSHES + TOOLS

_____

_____

_____

_____

NOTES

_____

_____

_____

_____

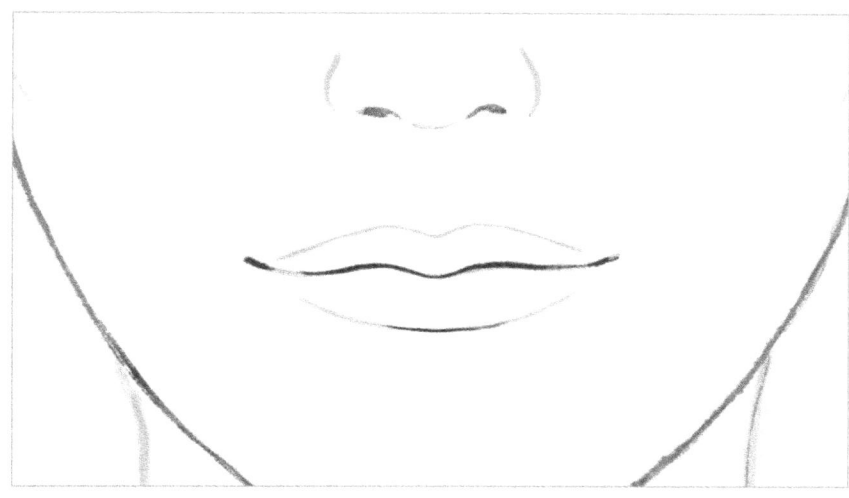

LOOK NAME_____

LIP SHAPE _Medium_____

LINER _____

COLOR _____

GLOSS _____

NOTES _____

_____

_____

_____

_____

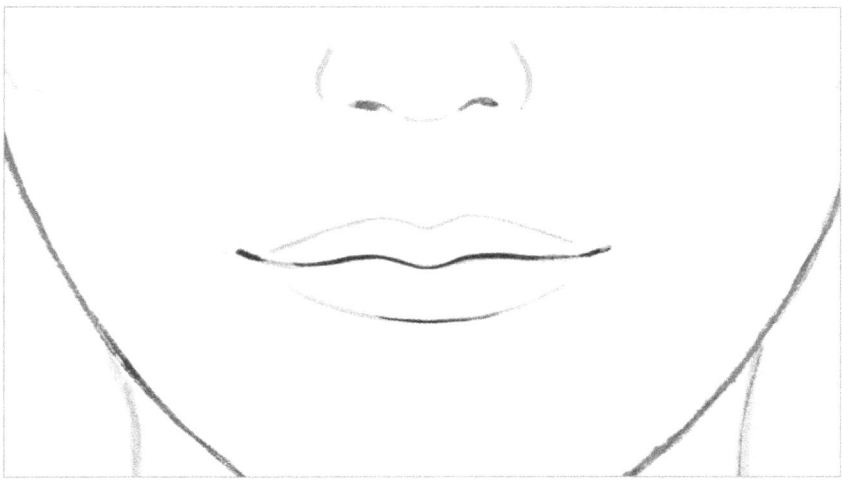

LOOK NAME_____

LIP SHAPE _Medium_____

LINER _____

COLOR _____

GLOSS _____

NOTES _____

_____

_____

_____

_____

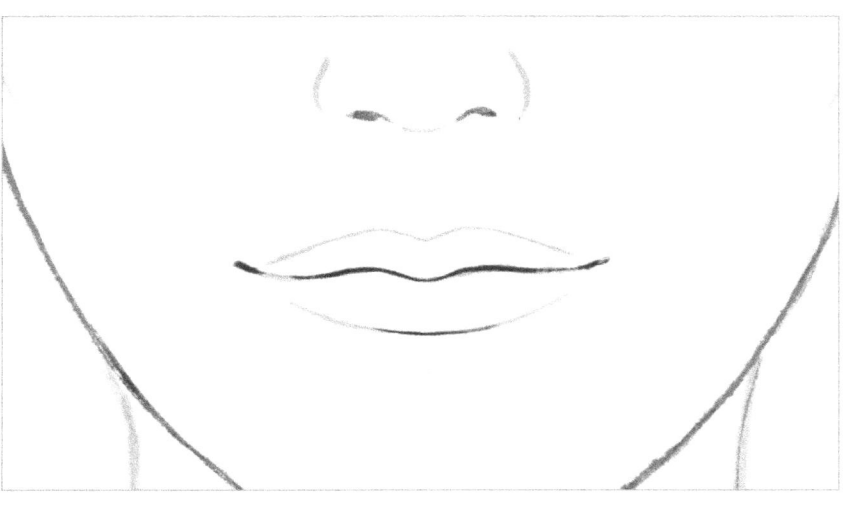

LOOK NAME_____

LIP SHAPE _Medium_____

LINER _____

COLOR _____

GLOSS _____

NOTES _____

_____

_____

_____

_____

BRUSHES + TOOLS

_____

_____

_____

_____

NOTES

_____

_____

_____

_____

BRUSHES + TOOLS

_____

_____

_____

_____

NOTES

_____

_____

_____

_____

BRUSHES + TOOLS

_____

_____

_____

_____

NOTES

_____

_____

_____

_____

makeup lip chart

LOOK NAME _____

LIP SHAPE <u>Medium</u>_____

LINER _____

COLOR _____

GLOSS _____

NOTES _____

CLIENT NAME _____

MAKEUP ARTIST _____

makeup lip chart

LOOK NAME _____

LIP SHAPE <u>Medium</u>_____

LINER _____

COLOR _____

GLOSS _____

NOTES _____

CLIENT NAME _____

MAKEUP ARTIST _____

BRUSHES + TOOLS

_____

_____

_____

NOTES

_____

_____

_____

BRUSHES + TOOLS

_____

_____

_____

NOTES

_____

_____

_____

makeup lip chart

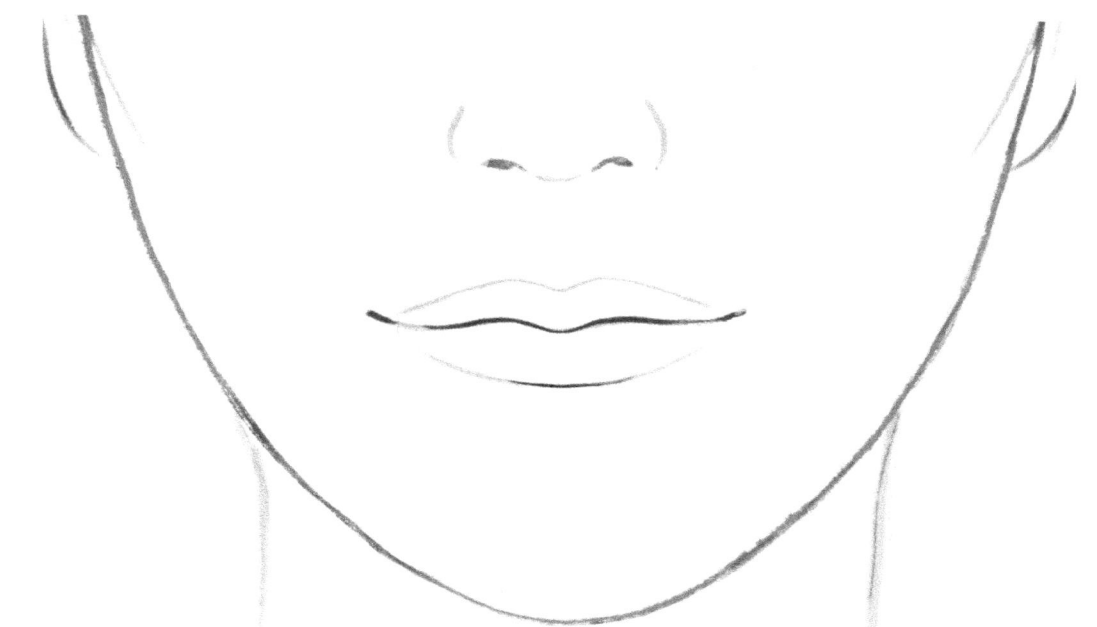

LOOK NAME _____

LIP SHAPE <u>Medium</u> _____

LINER _____

COLOR _____

GLOSS _____

NOTES _____

CLIENT NAME _____

MAKEUP ARTIST _____

makeup lip chart

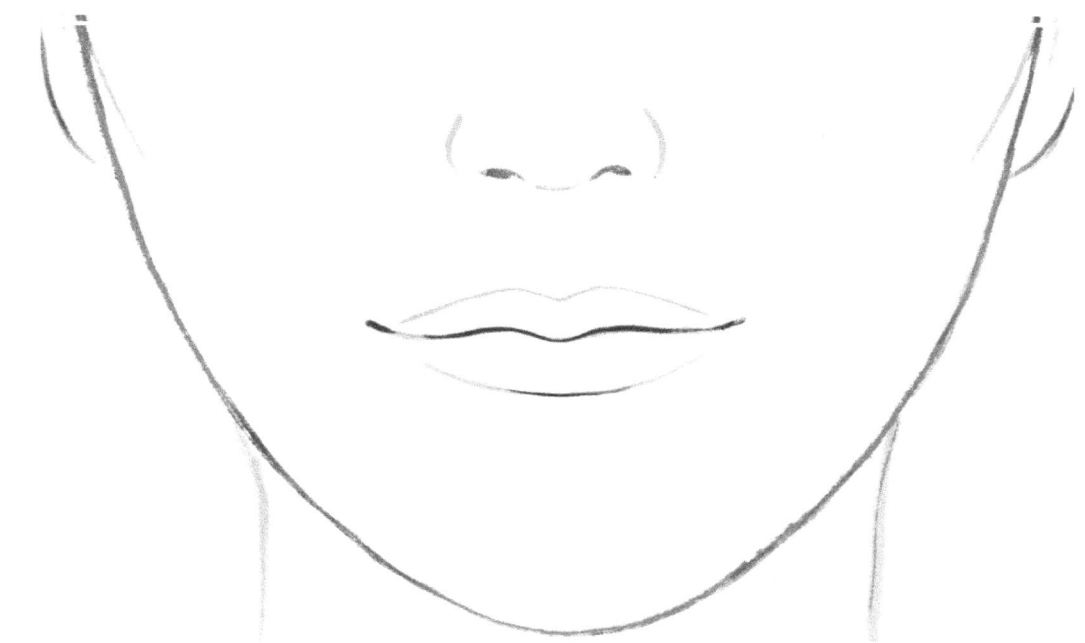

LOOK NAME _____

LIP SHAPE <u>Medium</u> _____

LINER _____

COLOR _____

GLOSS _____

NOTES _____

CLIENT NAME _____

MAKEUP ARTIST _____

BRUSHES + TOOLS

NOTES

_____

_____

_____

....

BRUSHES + TOOLS

NOTES

_____

_____

_____

makeup lip chart

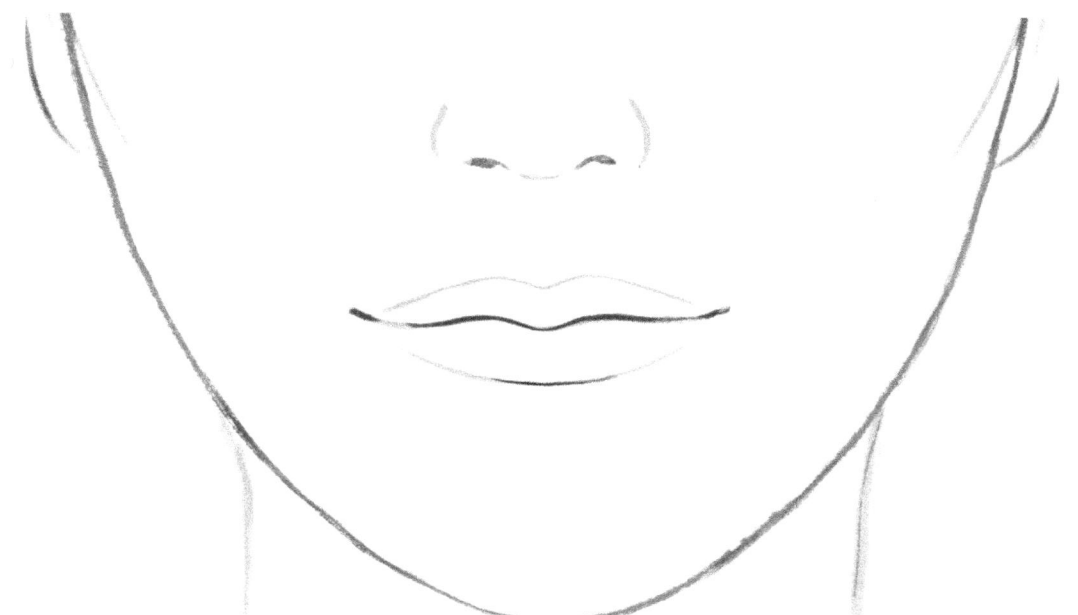

LOOK NAME _____

LIP SHAPE <u>Medium</u> _____

LINER _____

COLOR _____

GLOSS _____

NOTES _____

CLIENT NAME _____

MAKEUP ARTIST _____

makeup lip chart

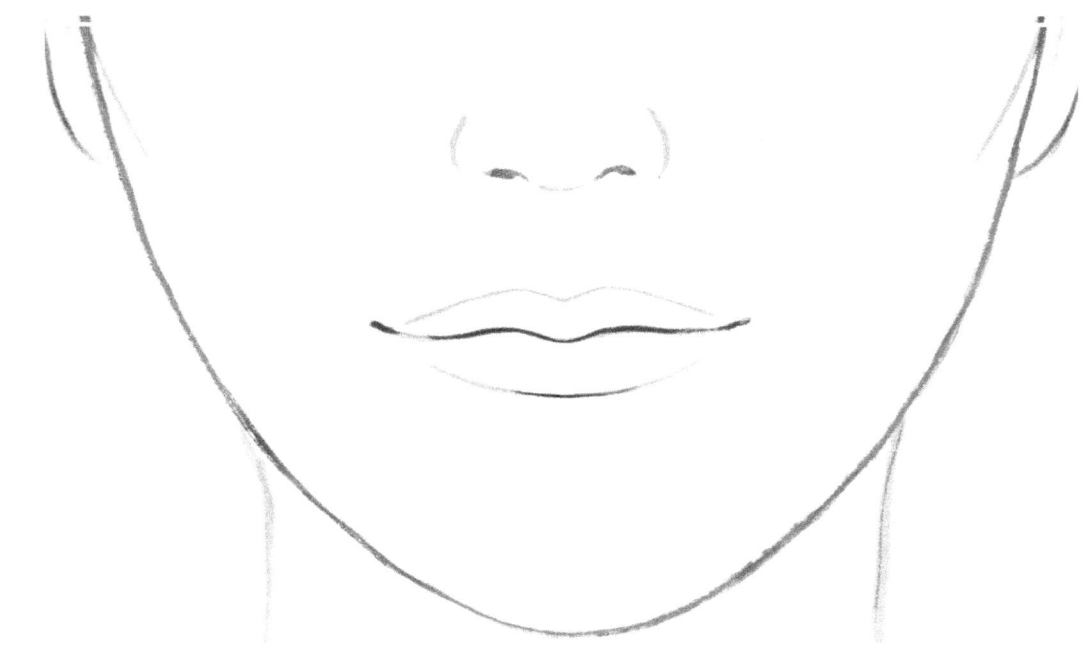

LOOK NAME _____

LIP SHAPE <u>Medium</u> _____

LINER _____

COLOR _____

GLOSS _____

NOTES _____

CLIENT NAME _____

MAKEUP ARTIST _____

BRUSHES + TOOLS

_____

_____

_____

NOTES

_____

_____

_____

BRUSHES + TOOLS

_____

_____

_____

NOTES

_____

_____

_____

makeup lip charts
Full Shape

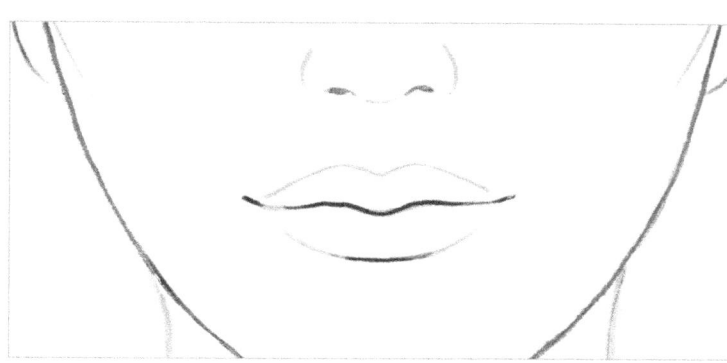

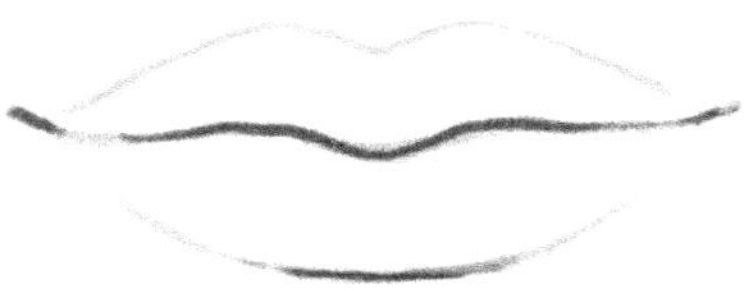

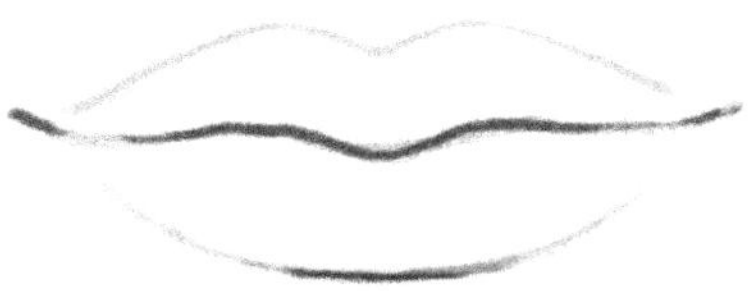

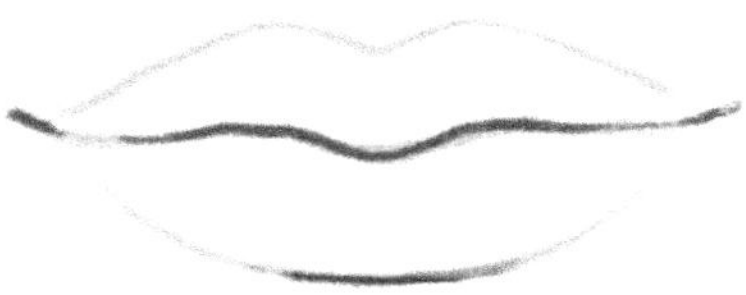

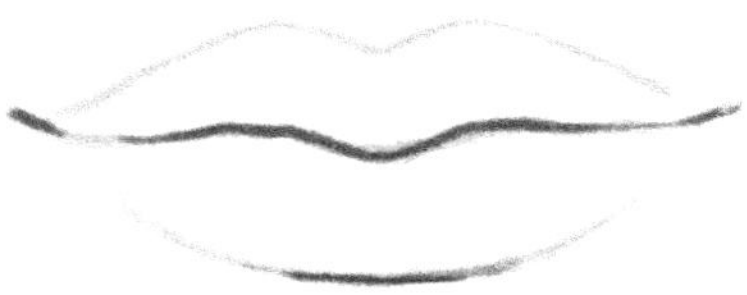

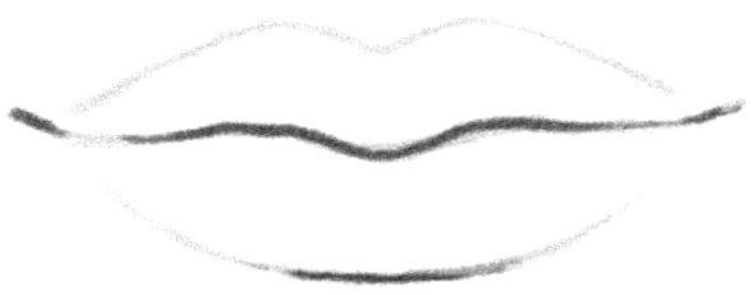

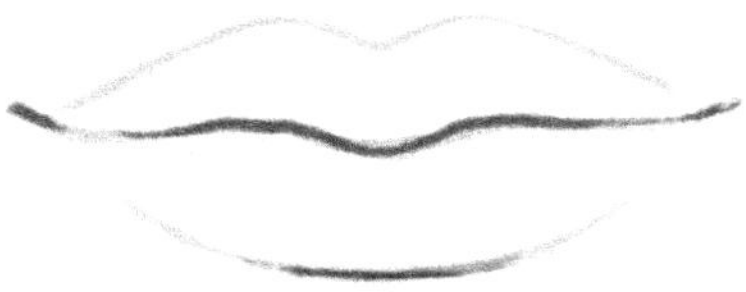

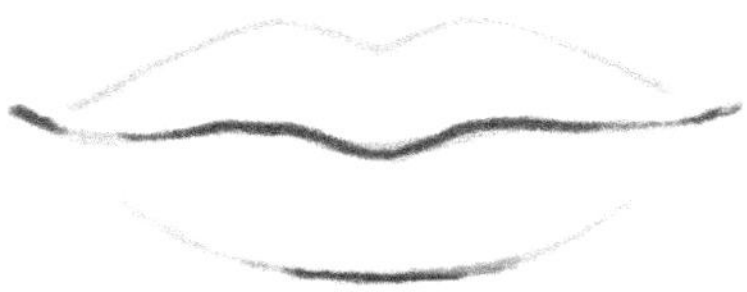

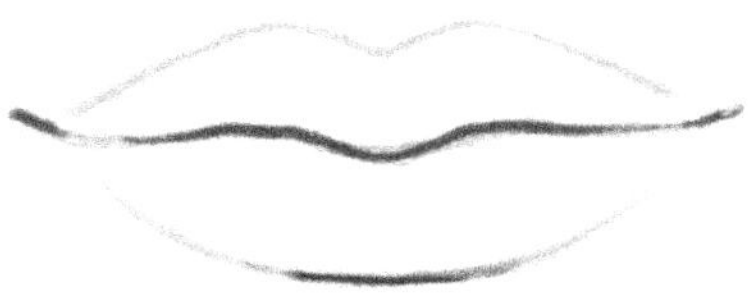

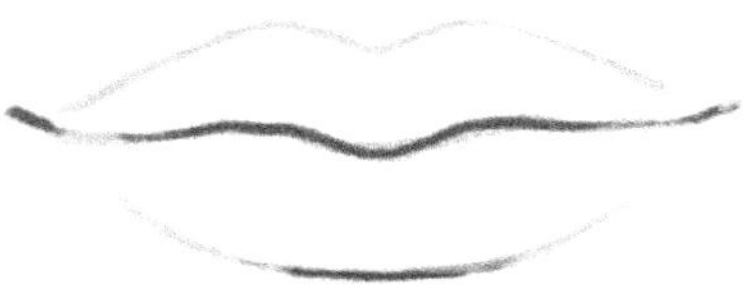

_____
_____
_____
_____

_____
_____
_____
_____

_____
_____
_____
_____

_____
_____
_____
_____

_____
_____
_____
_____

_____
_____
_____
_____

_____
_____
_____
_____

_____
_____
_____
_____

_____
_____
_____
_____

makeup lip charts

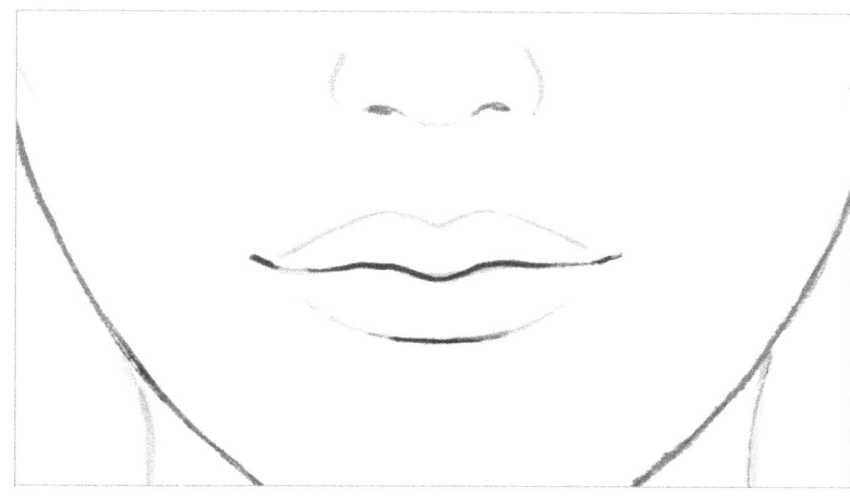

LOOK NAME_____

LIP SHAPE _Full_____

LINER _____

COLOR _____

GLOSS _____

NOTES _____

_____

_____

_____

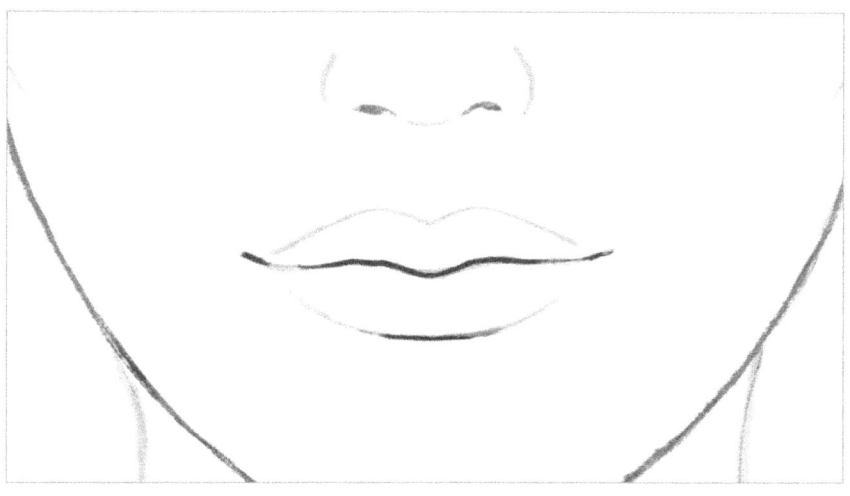

LOOK NAME_____

LIP SHAPE _Full_____

LINER _____

COLOR _____

GLOSS _____

NOTES _____

_____

_____

_____

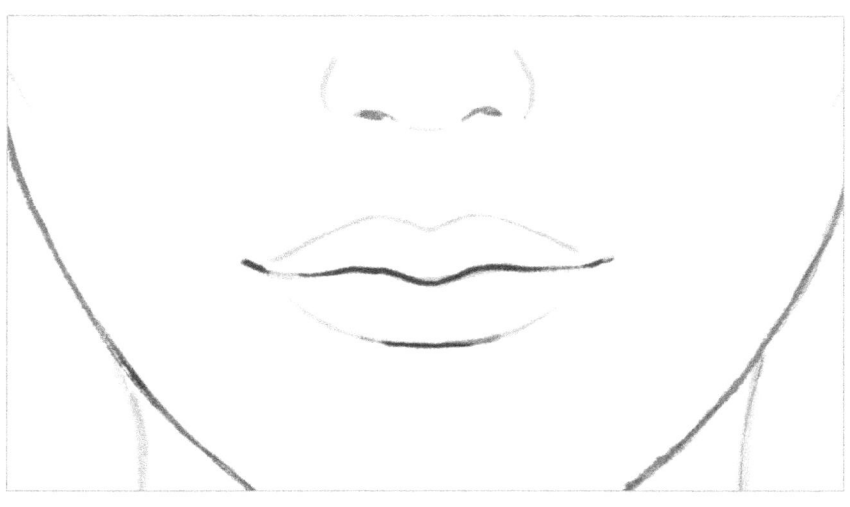

LOOK NAME_____

LIP SHAPE _Full_____

LINER _____

COLOR _____

GLOSS _____

NOTES _____

_____

_____

_____

BRUSHES + TOOLS

_____

_____

_____

_____

NOTES

_____

_____

_____

_____

BRUSHES + TOOLS

_____

_____

_____

_____

NOTES

_____

_____

_____

_____

BRUSHES + TOOLS

_____

_____

_____

_____

NOTES

_____

_____

_____

_____

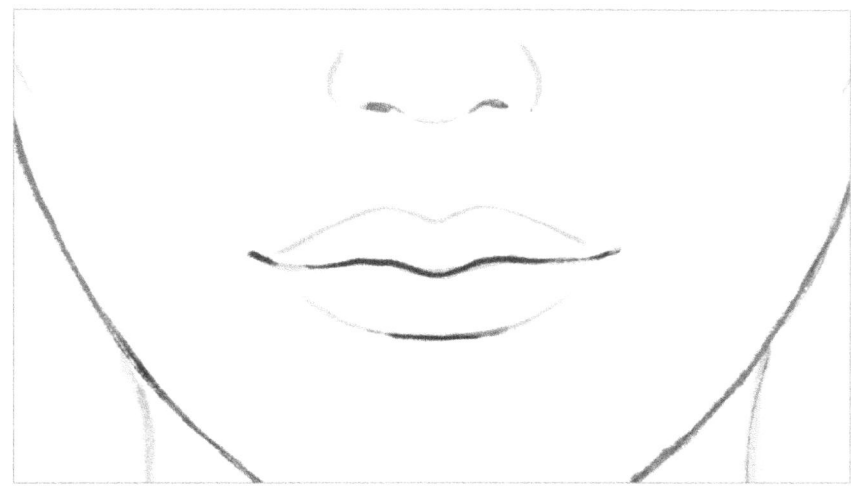

LOOK NAME_____

LIP SHAPE _Full_____

LINER _____

COLOR _____

GLOSS _____

NOTES _____

_____

_____

_____

_____

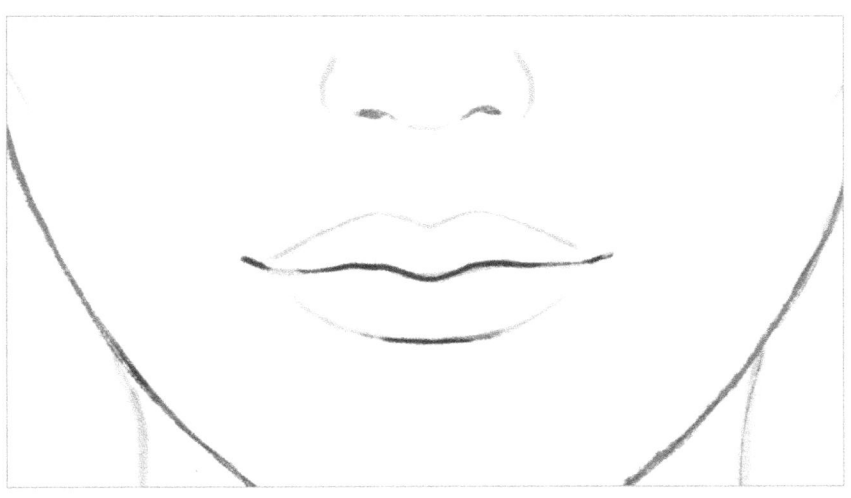

LOOK NAME_____

LIP SHAPE _Full_____

LINER _____

COLOR _____

GLOSS _____

NOTES _____

_____

_____

_____

_____

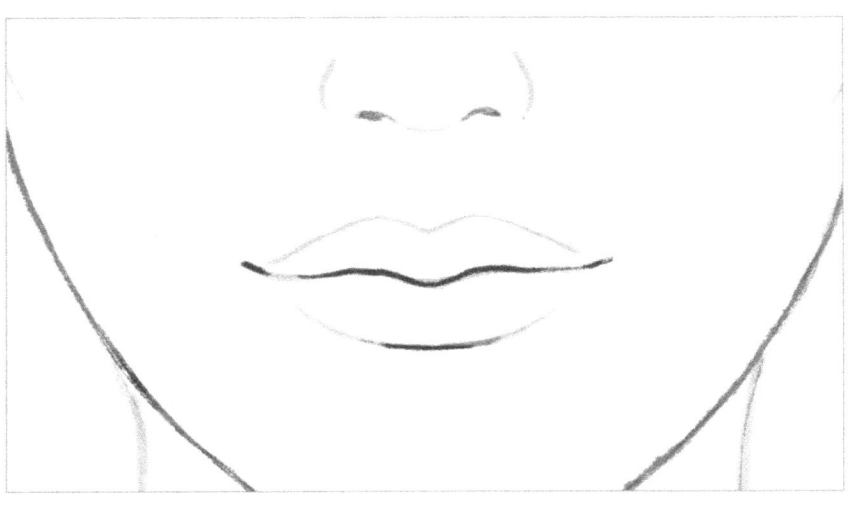

LOOK NAME_____

LIP SHAPE _Full_____

LINER _____

COLOR _____

GLOSS _____

NOTES _____

_____

_____

_____

_____

BRUSHES + TOOLS

_____

_____

_____

_____

NOTES

_____

_____

_____

_____

BRUSHES + TOOLS

_____

_____

_____

_____

NOTES

_____

_____

_____

_____

BRUSHES + TOOLS

_____

_____

_____

_____

NOTES

_____

_____

_____

_____

makeup lip chart

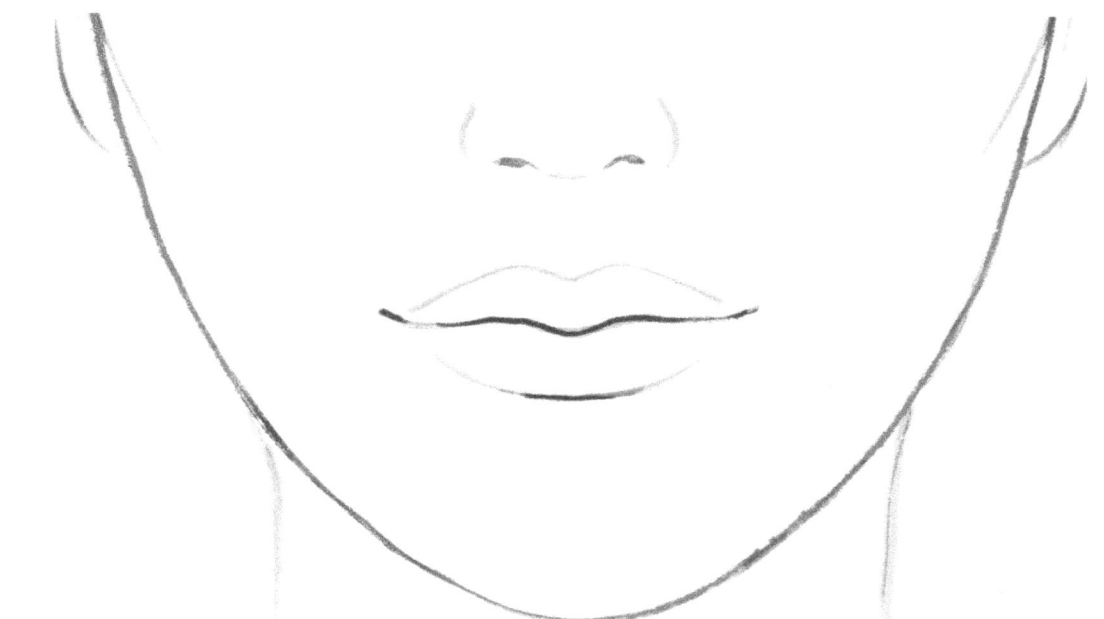

LOOK NAME _____

LIP SHAPE <u>Full</u> _____

LINER _____

COLOR _____

GLOSS _____

NOTES _____

CLIENT NAME _____

MAKEUP ARTIST _____

makeup lip chart

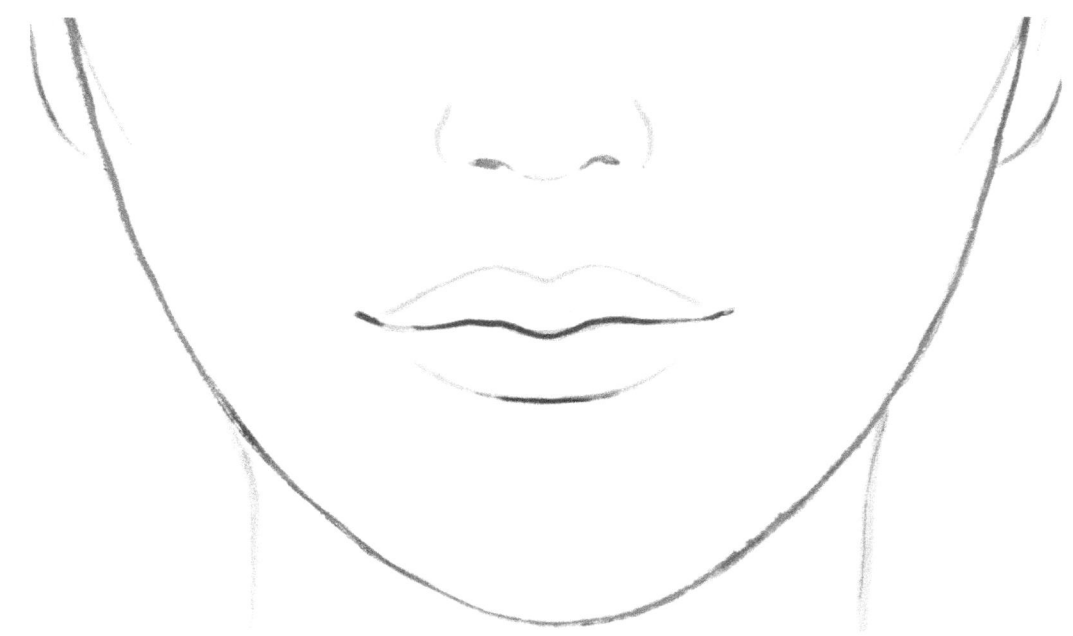

LOOK NAME _____

LIP SHAPE <u>Full</u> _____

LINER _____

COLOR _____

GLOSS _____

NOTES _____

CLIENT NAME _____

MAKEUP ARTIST _____

BRUSHES + TOOLS

_____

_____

_____

· ·

NOTES

_____

_____

_____

BRUSHES + TOOLS

_____

_____

_____

NOTES

_____

_____

_____

makeup lip chart

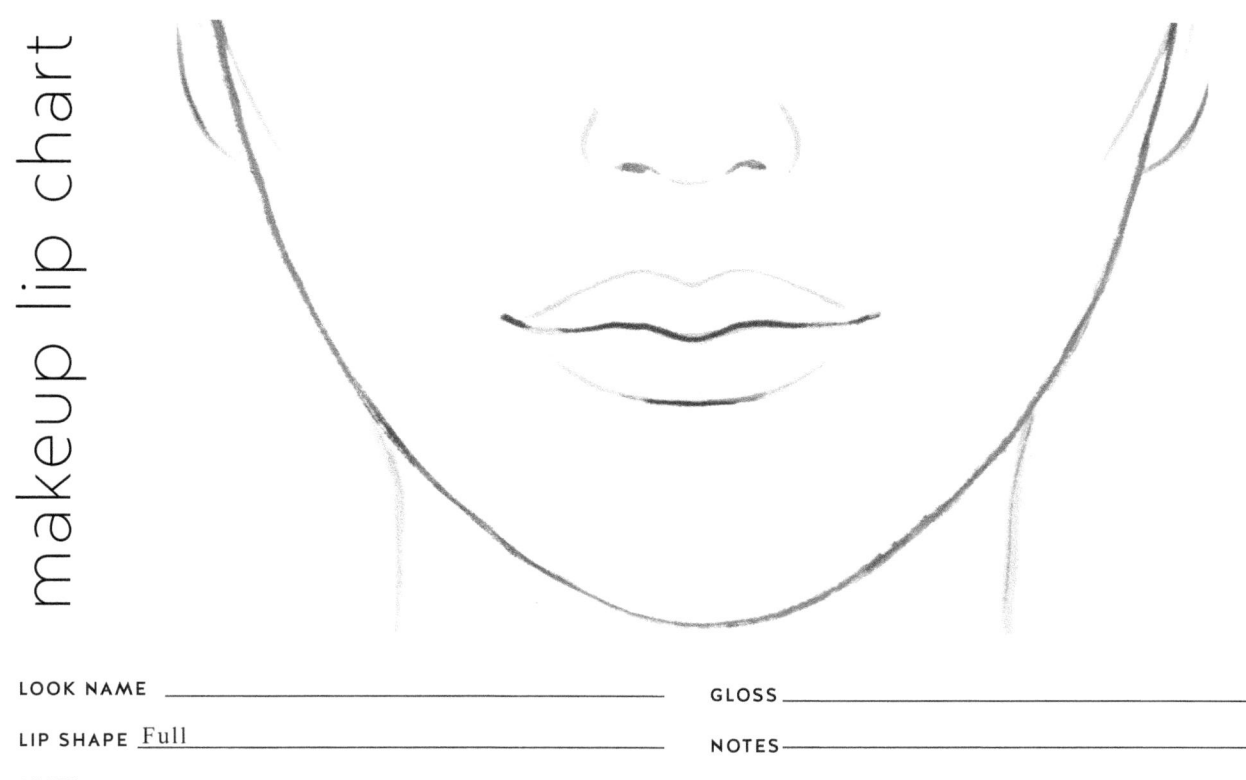

LOOK NAME _____

LIP SHAPE <u>Full</u> _____

LINER _____

COLOR _____

GLOSS _____

NOTES _____

CLIENT NAME _____

MAKEUP ARTIST _____

....

makeup lip chart

LOOK NAME _____

LIP SHAPE <u>Full</u> _____

LINER _____

COLOR _____

GLOSS _____

NOTES _____

CLIENT NAME _____

MAKEUP ARTIST _____

BRUSHES + TOOLS

_____

_____

_____

....

NOTES

_____

_____

_____

BRUSHES + TOOLS

_____

_____

_____

NOTES

_____

_____

_____

makeup lip chart

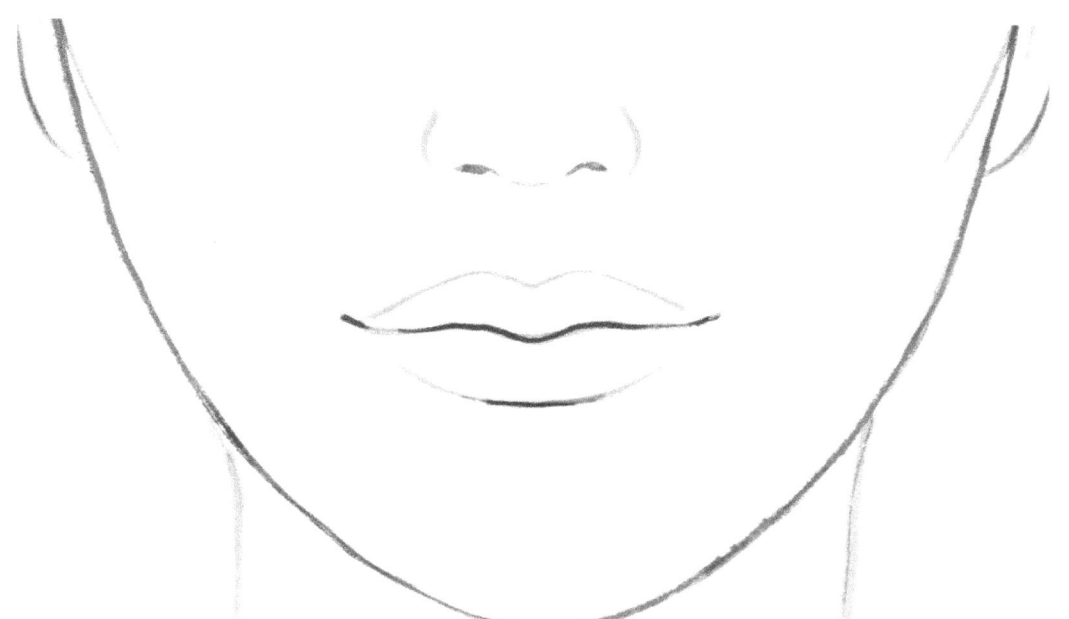

LOOK NAME _____

LIP SHAPE <u>Full</u> _____

LINER _____

COLOR _____

GLOSS _____

NOTES _____

CLIENT NAME _____

MAKEUP ARTIST _____

makeup lip chart

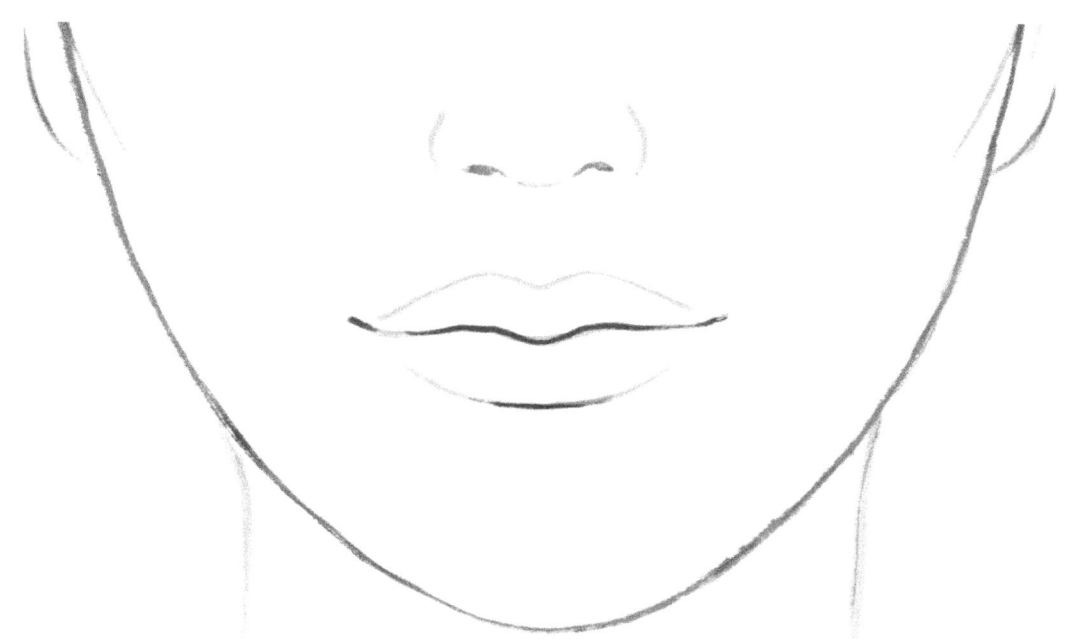

LOOK NAME _____

LIP SHAPE <u>Full</u> _____

LINER _____

COLOR _____

GLOSS _____

NOTES _____

CLIENT NAME _____

MAKEUP ARTIST _____

BRUSHES + TOOLS

_____

_____

_____

....

NOTES

_____

_____

_____

BRUSHES + TOOLS

_____

_____

_____

NOTES

_____

_____

_____

makeup lip charts
Extra-full Shape

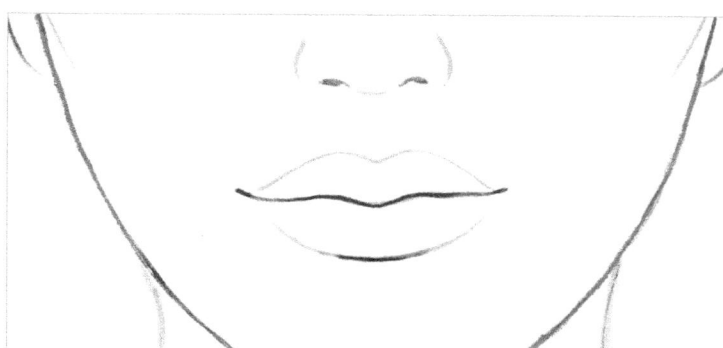

_____
_____
_____
_____

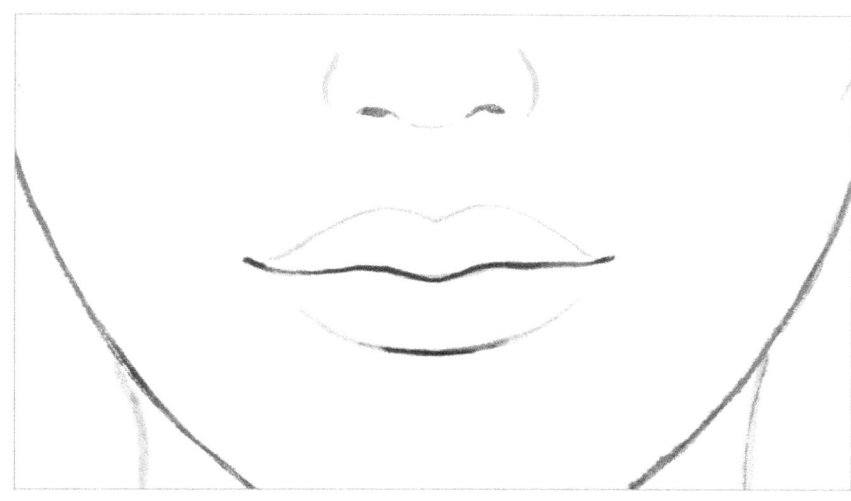

LOOK NAME_____

LIP SHAPE_Extra-full_____

LINER_____

COLOR_____

GLOSS_____

NOTES_____

_____

_____

_____

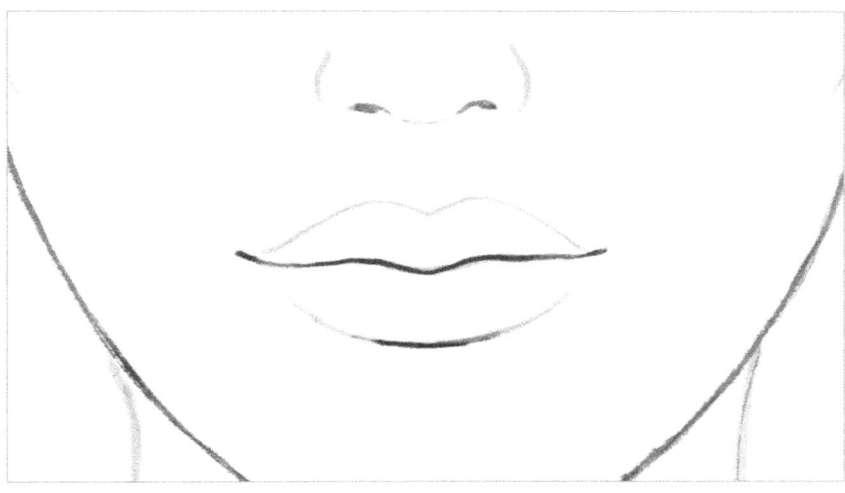

LOOK NAME_____

LIP SHAPE_Extra-full_____

LINER_____

COLOR_____

GLOSS_____

NOTES_____

_____

_____

_____

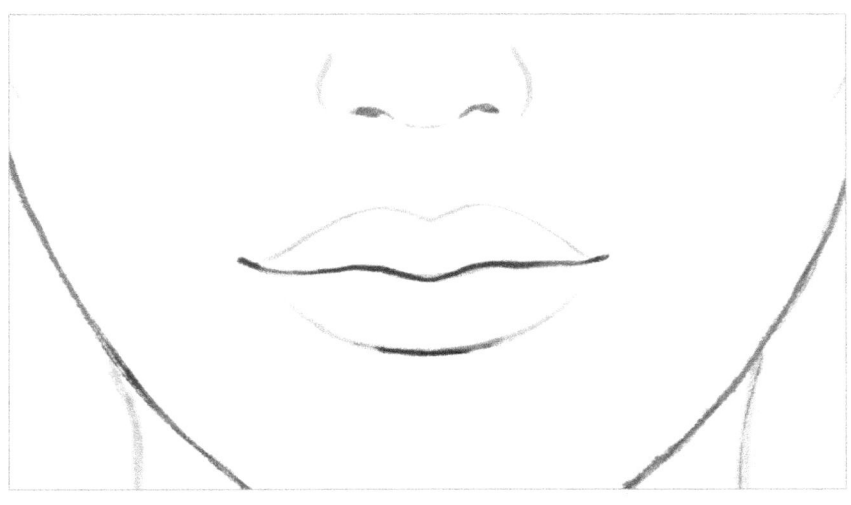

LOOK NAME_____

LIP SHAPE_Extra-full_____

LINER_____

COLOR_____

GLOSS_____

NOTES_____

_____

_____

_____

BRUSHES + TOOLS

_____

_____

_____

_____

NOTES

_____

_____

_____

_____

BRUSHES + TOOLS

_____

_____

_____

_____

NOTES

_____

_____

_____

_____

BRUSHES + TOOLS

_____

_____

_____

_____

NOTES

_____

_____

_____

_____

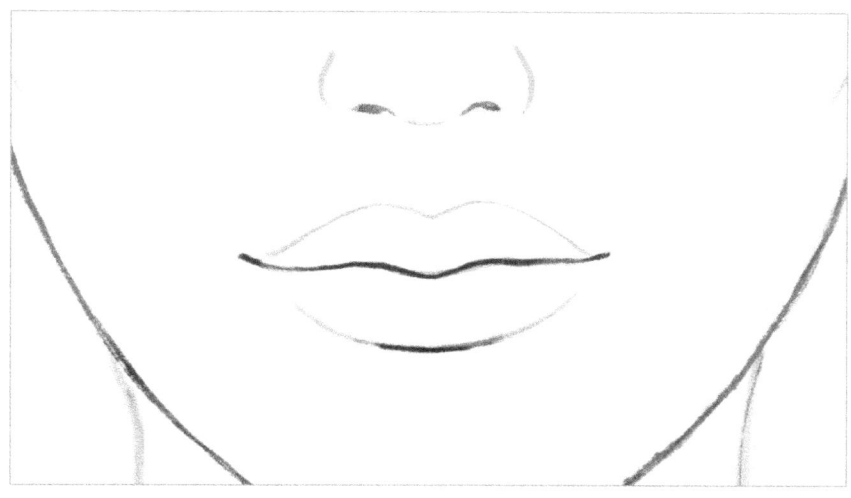

LOOK NAME _____

LIP SHAPE _Extra-full_____

LINER _____

COLOR _____

GLOSS _____

NOTES _____

_____

_____

_____

_____

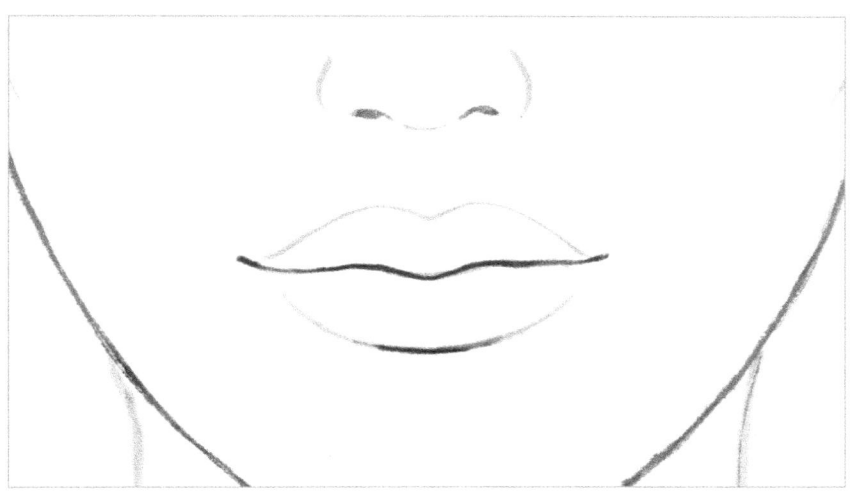

LOOK NAME _____

LIP SHAPE _Extra-full_____

LINER _____

COLOR _____

GLOSS _____

NOTES _____

_____

_____

_____

_____

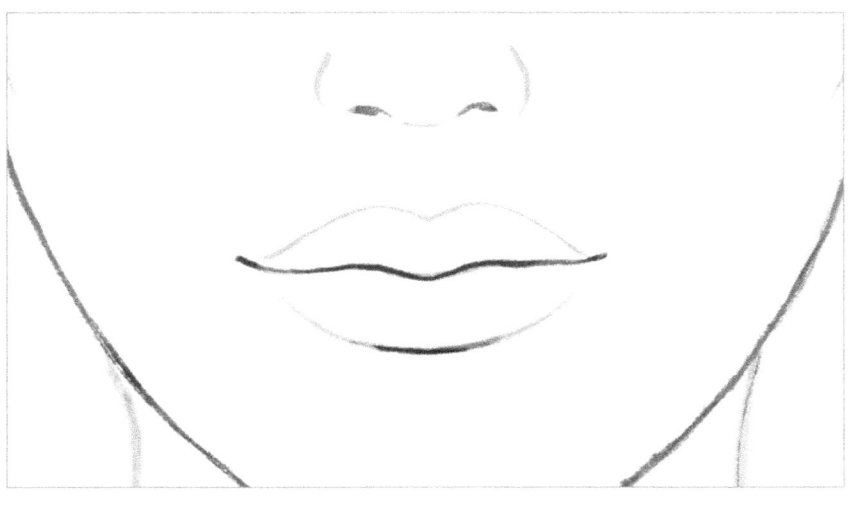

LOOK NAME _____

LIP SHAPE _Extra-full_____

LINER _____

COLOR _____

GLOSS _____

NOTES _____

_____

_____

_____

_____

BRUSHES + TOOLS

_____

_____

_____

_____

NOTES

_____

_____

_____

_____

....

BRUSHES + TOOLS

_____

_____

_____

_____

NOTES

_____

_____

_____

_____

....

BRUSHES + TOOLS

_____

_____

_____

_____

NOTES

_____

_____

_____

_____

makeup lip chart

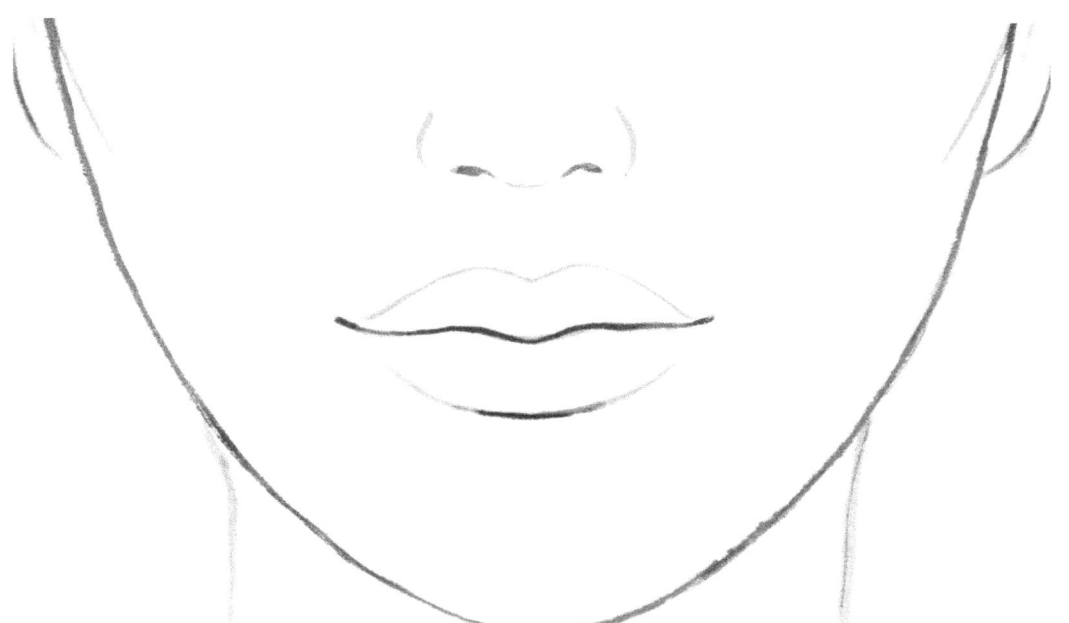

LOOK NAME _____

LIP SHAPE Extra-full _____

LINER _____

COLOR _____

GLOSS _____

NOTES _____

CLIENT NAME _____

MAKEUP ARTIST _____

makeup lip chart

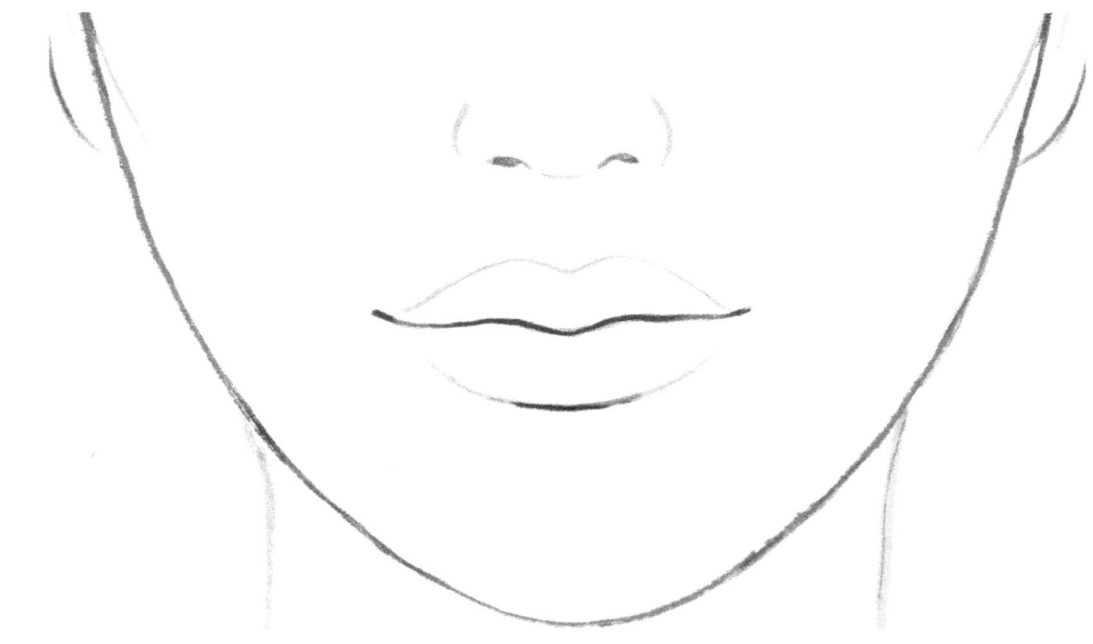

LOOK NAME _____

LIP SHAPE Extra-full _____

LINER _____

COLOR _____

GLOSS _____

NOTES _____

CLIENT NAME _____

MAKEUP ARTIST _____

BRUSHES + TOOLS

_____

_____

_____

NOTES

_____

_____

_____

BRUSHES + TOOLS

_____

_____

_____

NOTES

_____

_____

_____

makeup lip chart

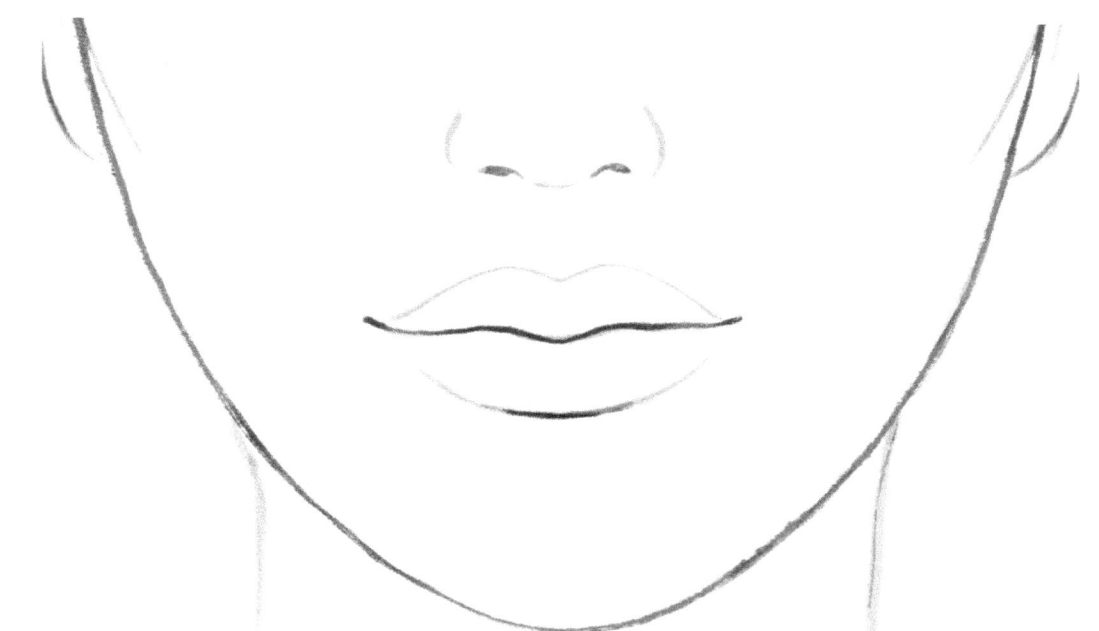

LOOK NAME _____

LIP SHAPE <u>Extra-full</u> _____

LINER _____

COLOR _____

GLOSS _____

NOTES _____

CLIENT NAME _____

MAKEUP ARTIST _____

---

makeup lip chart

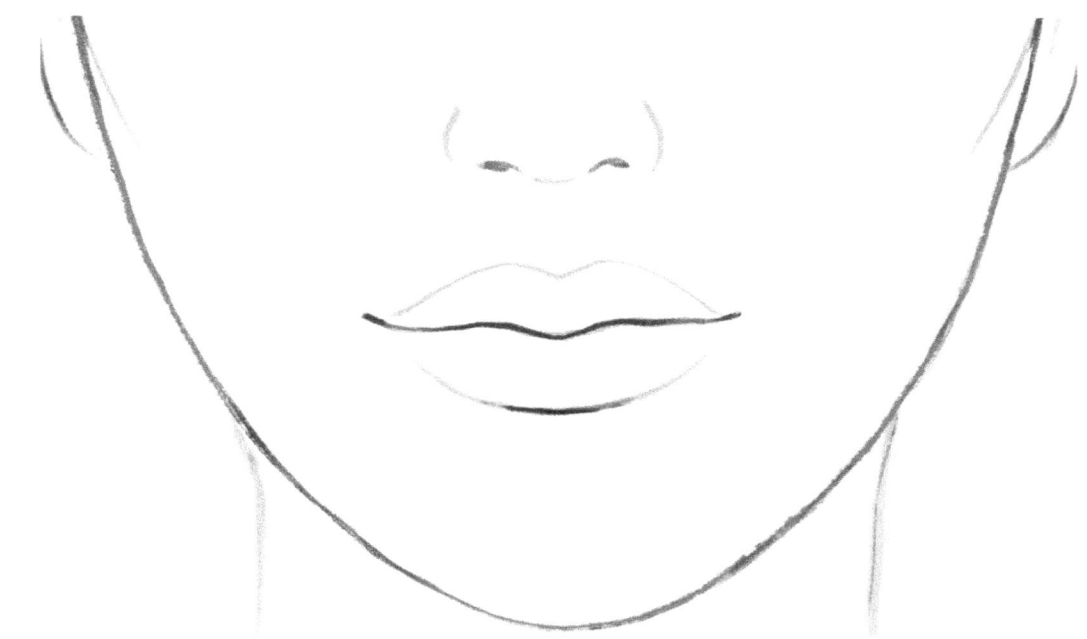

LOOK NAME _____

LIP SHAPE <u>Extra-full</u> _____

LINER _____

COLOR _____

GLOSS _____

NOTES _____

CLIENT NAME _____

MAKEUP ARTIST _____

BRUSHES + TOOLS

_____

_____

_____

· ·

NOTES

_____

_____

_____

BRUSHES + TOOLS

_____

_____

_____

NOTES

_____

_____

_____

makeup eye charts
Almond Shape

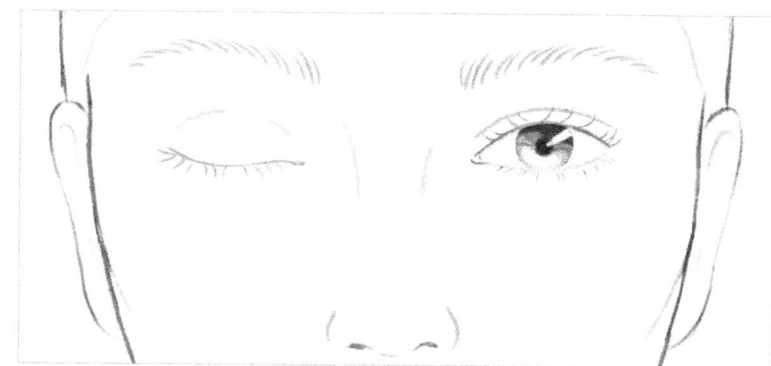

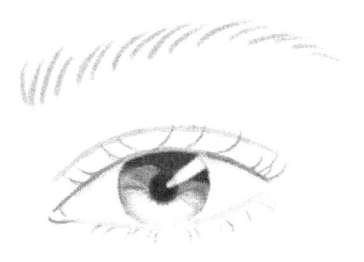

_____

_____

_____

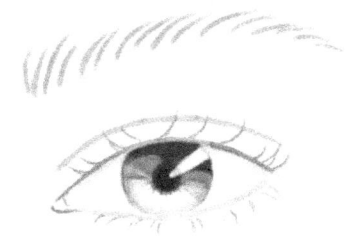

_____

_____

_____

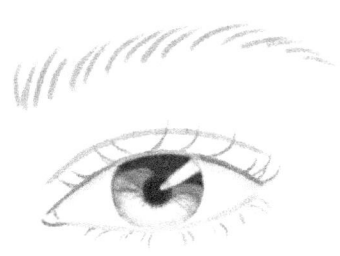

_____

_____

_____

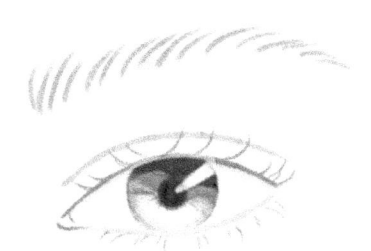

_____

_____

_____

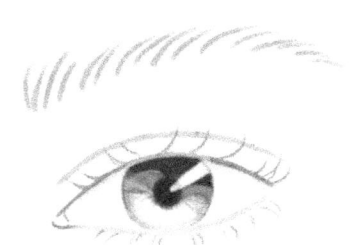

_____

_____

_____

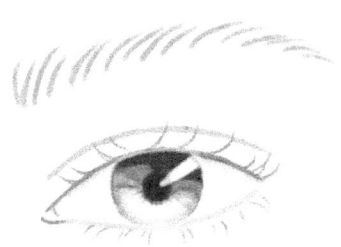

_____

_____

_____

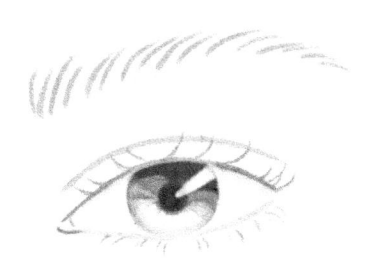

_____

_____

_____

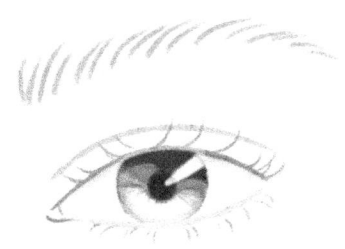

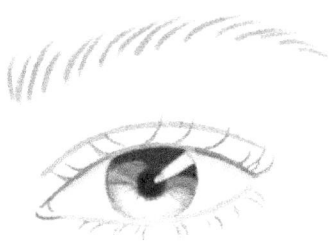

_____

_____

_____

LOOK NAME_____

EYE SHAPE _Almond_____

BROWS _____

LINER _____

EYE SHADOW _____

_____

LASHES _____

LOOK NAME_____

EYE SHAPE _Asian_____

BROWS _____

LINER _____

EYE SHADOW _____

_____

LASHES _____

LOOK NAME_____

EYE SHAPE _Round_____

BROWS _____

LINER _____

EYE SHADOW _____

_____

LASHES _____

LOOK NAME_____

EYE SHAPE _Hooded_____

BROWS _____

LINER _____

EYE SHADOW _____

_____

LASHES _____

BRUSHES + TOOLS

_____

_____

_____

_____

NOTES

_____

_____

_____

_____

BRUSHES + TOOLS

_____

_____

_____

_____

NOTES

_____

_____

_____

_____

BRUSHES + TOOLS

_____

_____

_____

_____

NOTES

_____

_____

_____

_____

BRUSHES + TOOLS

_____

_____

_____

_____

NOTES

_____

_____

_____

_____

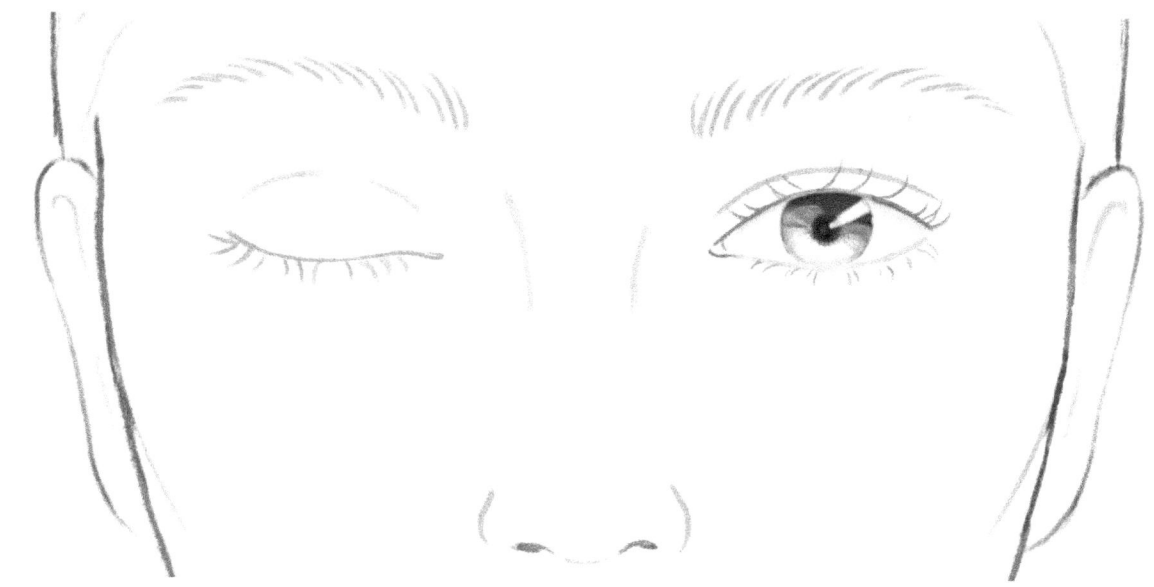

makeup eye chart

LOOK NAME _____

EYE SHAPE _Almond_____

BROWS _____

EYESHADOW_____

_____

MASCARA_____

LASHES_____

NOTES_____

CLIENT NAME _____

MAKEUP ARTIST _____

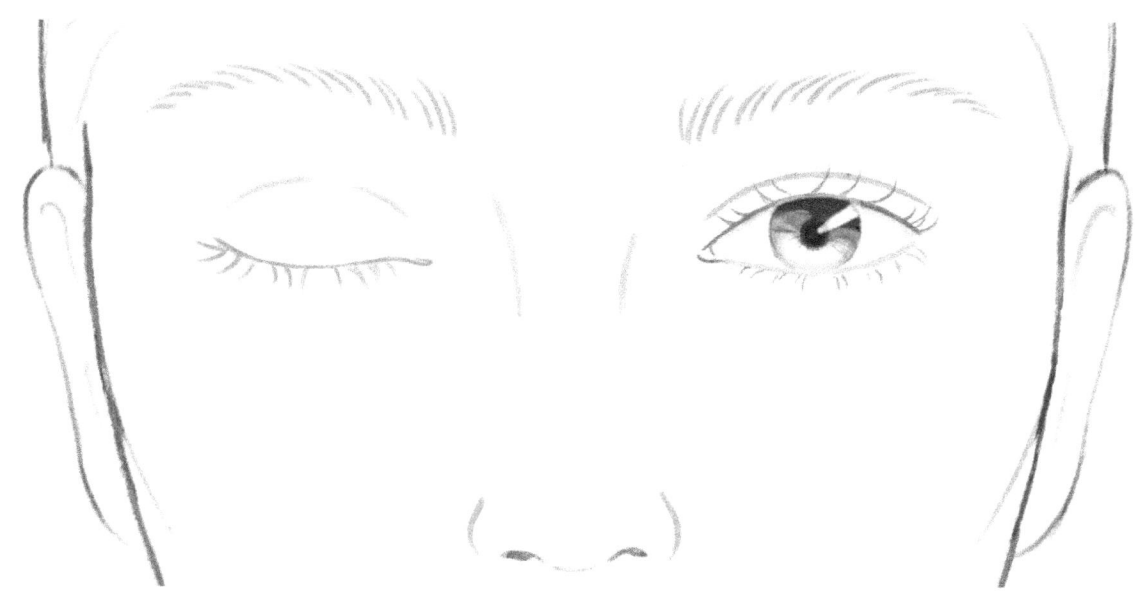

makeup eye chart

LOOK NAME _____

EYE SHAPE _Almond_____

BROWS _____

EYESHADOW_____

_____

MASCARA_____

LASHES_____

NOTES_____

CLIENT NAME _____

MAKEUP ARTIST_____

BRUSHES + TOOLS

_____

_____

_____

_____

NOTES

_____

_____

_____

_____

BRUSHES + TOOLS

_____

_____

_____

_____

NOTES

_____

_____

_____

_____

makeup brow charts

NAME _____

BROW SHAPE _Straight_____

_____

_____

_____

NAME _____

BROW SHAPE _Round_____

_____

_____

_____

NAME _____

BROW SHAPE _Soft Angle_____

_____

_____

_____

NAME _____

BROW SHAPE _Sharp Angle____

_____

_____

_____

NAME _____

BROW SHAPE _S-shape_____

_____

_____

makeup face chart

LOOK NAME

_____

EYES

Brows:_____

Base:_____

Eye shadow:_____

_____

_____

Eyeliner:_____

Mascara:_____

Lashes:_____

FACE

Primer: _____

Concealer: _____

Foundation:_____

Powder:_____

Blush: _____

Bronzer:_____

Contour: _____

Highlight:_____

LIPS

Liner:_____

Gloss:_____

Color:_____

_____

CLIENT NAME

_____

MAKEUP ARTIST

_____

BRUSHES + TOOLS

_____

_____

_____

_____

_____

NOTES

_____

_____

_____

_____

_____

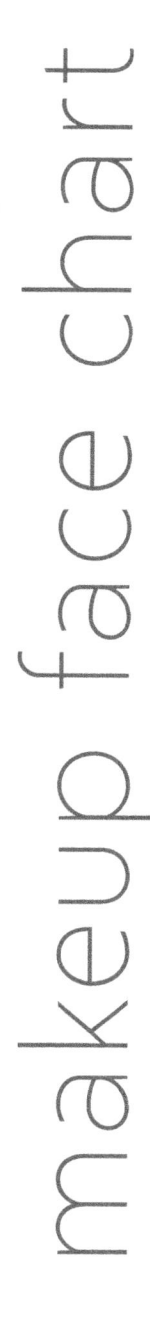

makeup face chart

LOOK NAME

_____

EYES

Brows:_____

Base:_____

Eye shadow:_____

_____

_____

Eyeliner:_____

Mascara:_____

Lashes:_____

FACE

Primer: _____

Concealer: _____

Foundation:_____

Powder:_____

Blush: _____

Bronzer: _____

Contour: _____

Highlight:_____

LIPS

Liner:_____

Gloss:_____

Color:_____

_____

CLIENT NAME

_____

MAKEUP ARTIST

_____

BRUSHES + TOOLS

_____

_____

_____

_____

_____

NOTES

_____

_____

_____

_____

_____

makeup face chart

LOOK NAME

_____

EYES

Brows:_____

Base:_____

Eye shadow:_____

_____

_____

Eyeliner:_____

Mascara:_____

Lashes:_____

FACE

Primer: _____

Concealer: _____

Foundation:_____

Powder:_____

Blush:_____

Bronzer:_____

Contour:_____

Highlight:_____

LIPS

Liner:_____

Gloss:_____

Color:_____

_____

CLIENT NAME

_____

MAKEUP ARTIST

_____

BRUSHES + TOOLS

_____

_____

_____

_____

_____

NOTES

_____

_____

_____

_____

_____

makeup face chart

LOOK NAME

_____

EYES

Brows:_____

Base:_____

Eye shadow:_____

_____

_____

Eyeliner:_____

Mascara:_____

Lashes:_____

FACE

Primer: _____

Concealer: _____

Foundation:_____

Powder:_____

Blush: _____

Bronzer: _____

Contour: _____

Highlight:_____

LIPS

Liner:_____

Gloss:_____

Color:_____

_____

CLIENT NAME

_____

MAKEUP ARTIST

_____

BRUSHES + TOOLS

_____

_____

_____

_____

_____

NOTES

_____

_____

_____

_____

_____

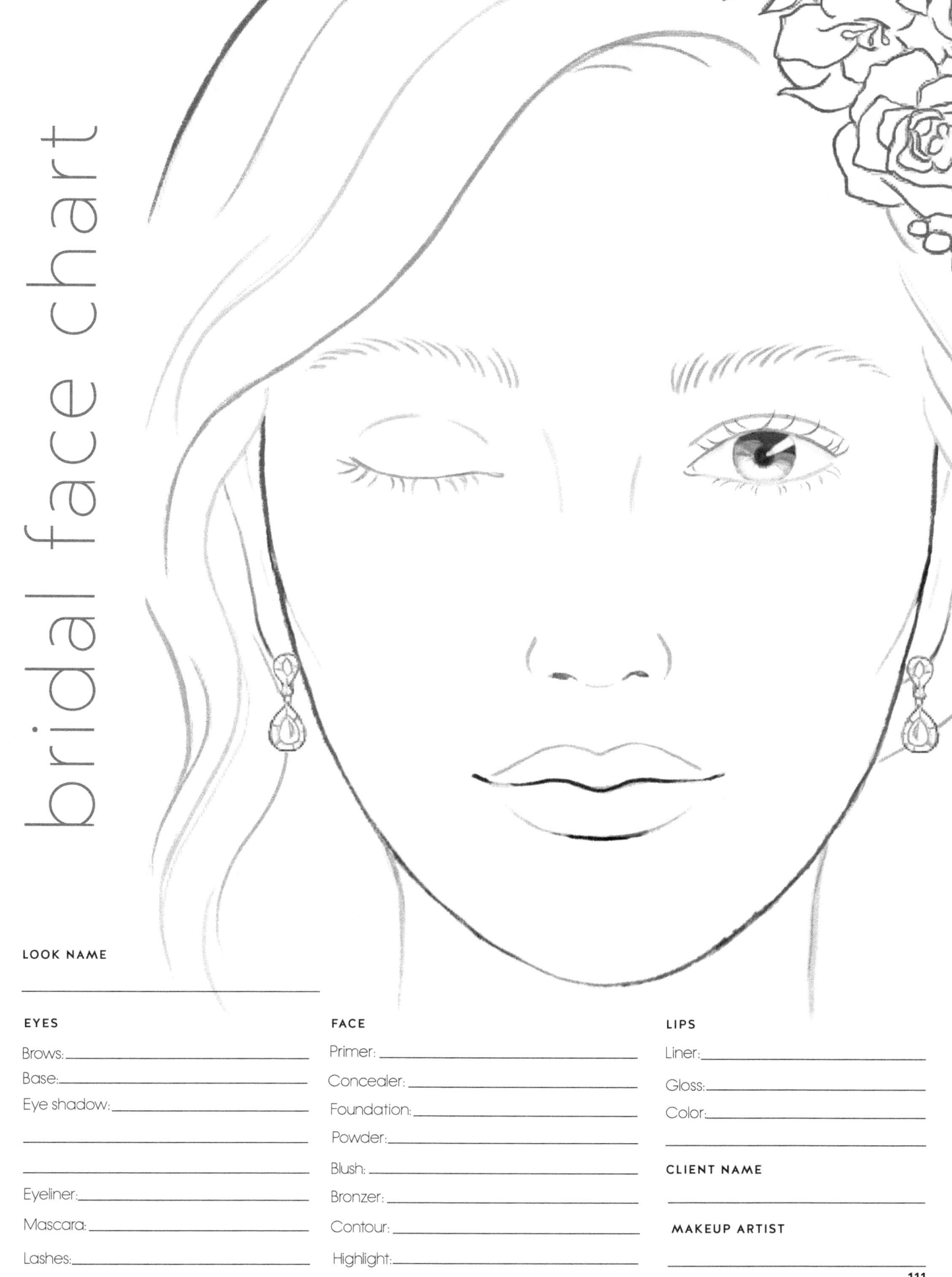

bridal face chart

LOOK NAME

_____

EYES

Brows:_____

Base:_____

Eye shadow:_____

_____

_____

Eyeliner:_____

Mascara:_____

Lashes:_____

FACE

Primer: _____

Concealer: _____

Foundation: _____

Powder:_____

Blush:_____

Bronzer: _____

Contour: _____

Highlight:_____

LIPS

Liner:_____

Gloss:_____

Color:_____

_____

CLIENT NAME

_____

MAKEUP ARTIST

_____

BRUSHES + TOOLS

_____

_____

_____

_____

_____

NOTES

_____

_____

_____

_____

_____

WEDDING DETAILS

_____

_____

_____

_____

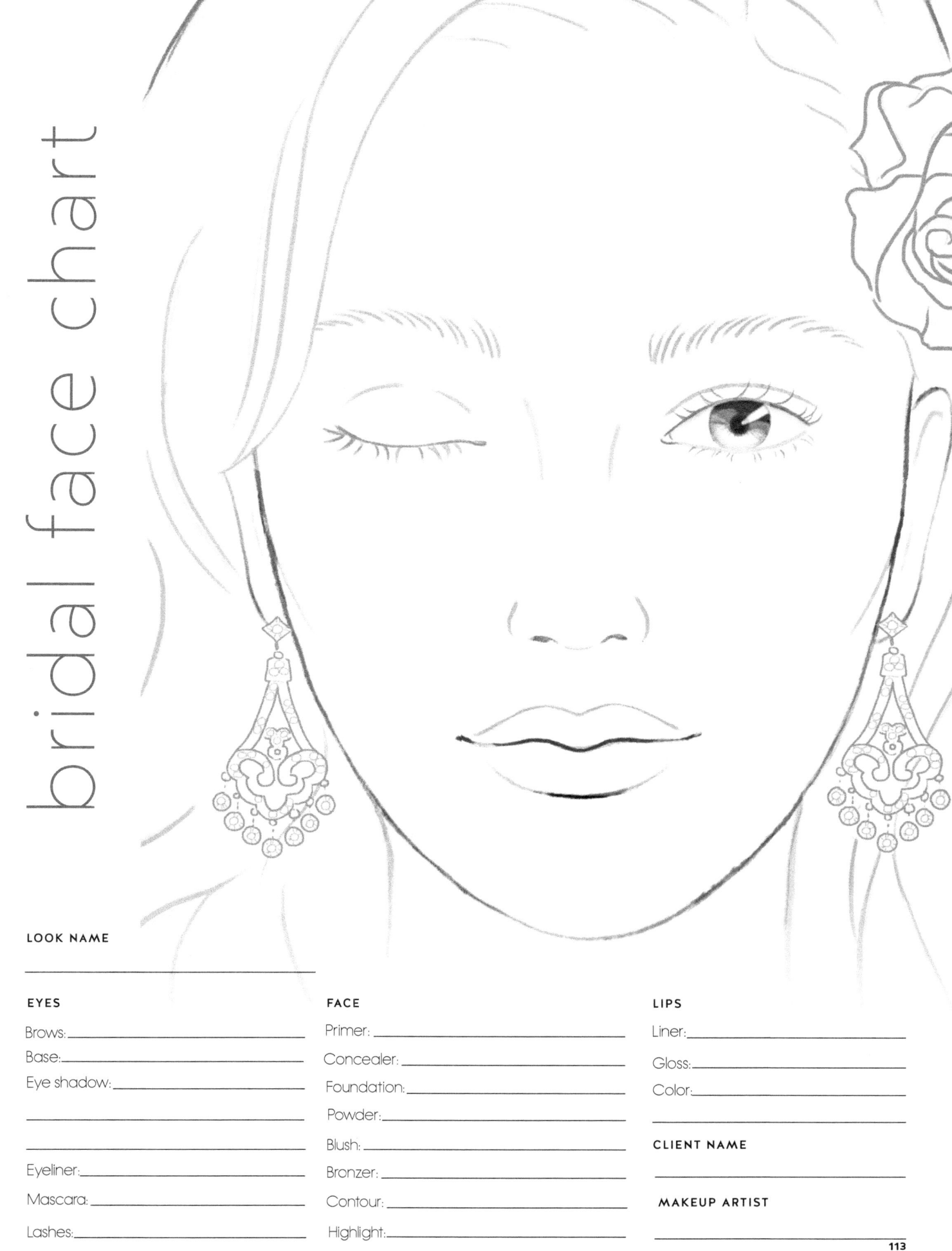

bridal face chart

LOOK NAME

_____

EYES

Brows:_____

Base:_____

Eye shadow:_____

_____

_____

Eyeliner:_____

Mascara:_____

Lashes:_____

FACE

Primer: _____

Concealer:_____

Foundation:_____

Powder:_____

Blush:_____

Bronzer: _____

Contour:_____

Highlight:_____

LIPS

Liner:_____

Gloss:_____

Color:_____

_____

CLIENT NAME

_____

MAKEUP ARTIST

_____

113

BRUSHES + TOOLS

_____

_____

_____

_____

_____

NOTES

_____

_____

_____

_____

_____

WEDDING DETAILS

_____

_____

_____

_____

Square Face Shape
HIGHLIGHT + CONTOUR GUIDE

The highlight and contouring method for a **Square** face shape focuses on lengthening to counter-balance width and round out sharp angles of the forehead and jaw.

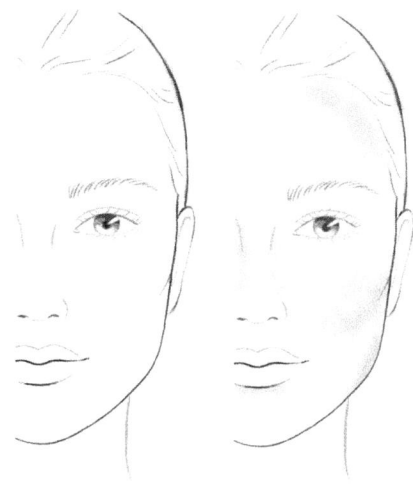

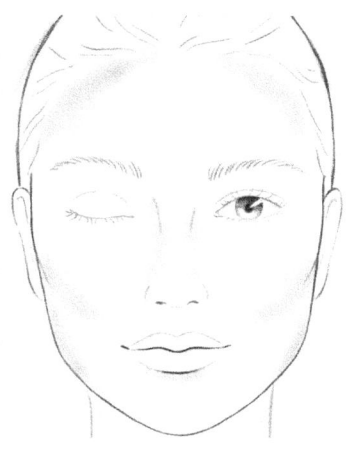

STEP 1: CONTOUR

Use dome blender brush and contour powder to shade:

Corners of forehead
Under cheekbones (curved line)
Sides of neck (optional)

Define shading on **corners of forehead & under cheekbones** with flat shader brush & contour powder.

Add shading to **sides of nose & under bottom lip** with pencil brush & contour powder. Also add contour along **jaw** to soften sharp angle.

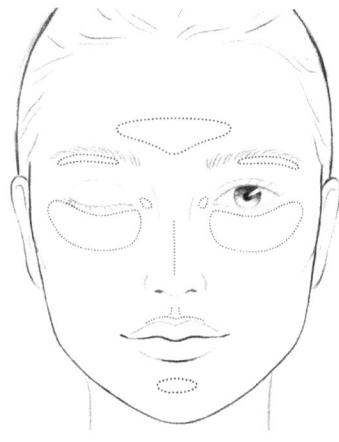

STEP 2: HIGHLIGHT + MID-TONE

Highlights are placed on the high points of the face. Use dome blender brush to apply highlight powder to (or leave areas blank if using white of paper as highlight)::

Forehead
Browbone
Inner eye corners
Under eyes
Cheekbones
Bridge of nose
Cupids bow
Center of chin

Apply mid-tone skincolor to blank areas between contour & highlight. Use small circular motions to create a seamless blend.

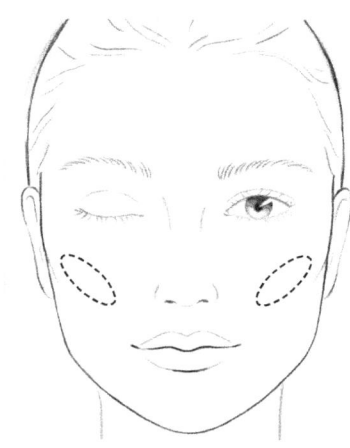

STEP 3: BLUSH

Elongate & lenghten by adding oval shading in upward diagnol.

Apply blush with blender brush for added shape and natural flush of color.

sculpt + shape chart

LOOK NAME _____

FACE SHAPE: <u>Square</u>_____

HIGHLIGHT _____

CONTOUR _____

MID-TONE _____

FACE _____

_____

_____

_____

EYES _____

_____

_____

_____

LIPS _____

_____

_____

BRUSHES + TOOLS

_____

_____

_____

_____

_____

NOTES

_____

_____

_____

_____

_____

About the Creator

Gina M. Reyna, founder and owner of Colorista Books, has been a professional makeup artist since 2009. She is an Empire Beauty School graduate & has attended fine art classes at the Art Institute and the Academy of Art University San Francisco. Her experience as a makeup artist ranges from weddings & special events to editorial-style photography.

When Gina isn't working as a makeup artist, she spends her time creating content for makeup artists and beauty enthusiasts. Her first book, 'How to be a Professional Makeup Artist - A Comprehensive Guide for Beginners', was published in January of 2013. She has since then written 'The Complete Guide to Smokey Eyes' & created The Beauty Studio Collection of makeup charts.

If you have a question or comment for Gina, please send it to: gina@coloristabooks.com

To learn more visit us at:
COLORISTABOOKS.COM